CERTIFIED OPHTHALMIC MEDICAL TECHNOLOGIST EXAM REVIEW MANUAL

CERTIFIED OPHTHALMIC MEDICAL TECHNOLOGIST EXAM REVIEW MANUAL

Janice K. Ledford, COMT

EyeWrite Productions

Franklin, North Carolina

The Basic Bookshelf for Eyecare Professionals

Series Editors: Janice K. Ledford, COMT   Ken Daniels, OD   Robert Campbell, MD

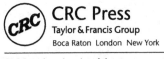

CRC Press
Taylor & Francis Group
Boca Raton London New York

CRC Press is an imprint of the
Taylor & Francis Group, an **informa** business

First published 1999 by SLACK Incorporated

Published 2024 by CRC Press
2385 NW Executive Center Drive, Suite 320, Boca Raton FL 33431

and by CRC Press
4 Park Square, Milton Park, Abingdon, Oxon, OX14 4RN

CRC Press is an imprint of Taylor & Francis Group, LLC

ISBN: 9781556424229 (hbk)
ISBN: 9781003522959 (ebk)

DOI: 10.1201/9781003522959

Dedication

To my husband, Jim, as we approach 25 years together.

1. Which of the following apply to Jim Ledford?

    a) He's a great guy

    b) He's a good cook

    c) He puts up with me and my writing

    d) All of the above

1. d) Only possible answer, of course.

Contents

Acknowledgments

Once again, there is a whole list of wonderful people who helped me on my way as I wrote this book. First, thanks to my editor, Dr. Bob Campbell, who had to go through the entire manuscript. That was no small task, believe me. Next, there was a fine group of professionals who were willing to review selected portions of the questions. Most are Series authors with books of their own. Without them, this book would not have come to be. Please understand that each of these folks is incredibly busy with his or her own patients and staff:

Charles Kirby, MD (microbiology, tonometry, pharmacology)

Gretchen Van Boemel, PhD, COMT (electrodiagnostics and other selected topics)

Neil Choplin, MD (visual fields . . . and finding other help!)

Peter Custis, MD (laser)

Barbara Brown, CO, COMT, MEd (low vision)

Denise Cunningham, COA, CRA, RBP, MEd (photography)

Al Lens, COMT (optics)

Scott McClatchey, MD (motility/strabismus)

I've had the pleasure of being associated with SLACK Incorporated for about 10 years now. This is the seventh book I've written for them . . . not to mention the 20-some-odd books I've edited for them, the manuscript reviews, and other stuff. At the risk of leaving anyone out, I'd like to thank these by name: Amy Drummond, John Bond, Debra Christy, Lauren Plummer, Vikki Kristiansson, Betsy DeBoer, and Jennifer Cahill. These people are the absolute best in the business.

Finally, without the support of my family, I wouldn't be a writer at all. My husband, Jim, is always glad to field general medical questions (which include "Honey, my sinuses are acting up again. What should I take?"). He is also very tolerant when he comes home from work and I'm still sitting at my computer, eyes glazed and fingers flying, with no idea what's for supper. (Perhaps he's become such a good cook out of self-defense?!?) The boys are also very understanding when I get the "crazies" just before the deadline of a big project. TJ managed to graduate *from* high school and Collin has managed to make it *to* high school in spite of it. And even the cats give an assist by helping me eat my snacks, watching faxes come out of the machine, chasing the cursor on the computer monitor, and keeping my chair warm any time I get up.

Yep, this writing thing is definitely a group effort. And what a group! I thank you sincerely, one and all.

About the Author

What to say about author Jan Ledford? "I've been around a long time!" she laughs. Jan started her journey in ophthalmology in 1982, 2 years after obtaining associate's degrees in dental hygiene and general studies (emphasis biology) from Columbus College in Columbus, Ga. How did she go from the mouth to the eye? She shrugs and says, "I needed a job."

It turned out to be more than a job . . . it turned into a career that has spanned 17 years and all three certification levels (COA in 1983, COT in 1984, and COMT in 1988). That experience helped prompt her to write the exam review books for all three levels. "Studying on my own for those exams gave me a real heart for others doing the same thing," she says. "And I believe in being the best you possibly can be. To me, that means getting certified."

Jan's clinical experience has been varied. She spent the first 3 years of her career (1982 to 1985) with Dr. George Hubbard in Columbus. "He was a great teacher, and expected a lot from his techs. When he interviewed me, he told me 'We only hire superstars here.' I looked him in the eye and said, 'Good. I should fit right in.' Now I can't believe I was that bold, or that I got the job anyway! It was a great place to start my career. Back then, almost nothing was automated. I learned everything from the ground up." By the time she left Columbus, she was a COT and the practice's continuing education coordinator. But just before leaving, another key event occurred: her first ophthalmic-related article was accepted for publication in *The Journal of Ophthalmic Nursing and Technology*. "That didn't just give off a spark," she says. "It lit a fire."

From 1985 to 1992, and again from 1994 to 1996, Jan worked for Dr. Johnny Gayton at Eye sight Associates of Middle Georgia in Warner Robins, Ga. Their long association began with a return to her hometown, where both she and her husband had grown up. "Two important things happened there," she says. "First, I was encouraged to get my COMT. Second, Dr. Gayton noticed my knack for writing and pressed me to use it." During her tenure there, she had 28 articles published. Some were written for Dr. Gayton (who thus appears as first author), but most on her own. Journals that have published her work include *Ophthalmology, Ophthalmology World News, Annals of Ophthalmology and Glaucoma, Contact Lens Spectrum, Ophthalmic Plastic and Reconstructive Surgery, Phaco & Foldables*, and the *Journal of the Medical Association of Georgia*. She wrote numerous pamphlets and audio scripts for patient education purposes, as well as an eyecare column and other newspaper articles. Eventually she expanded from articles to books, authoring SLACK's *Exercises in Refractometry* (1990) and *In-Office Training Manual and Series Review* (1992).

During this time she founded her own company, EyeWrite Productions, for the specific purpose of writing and editing material in the eyecare field. "The next step seemed obvious," she notes. "One day, Dr. Gayton passed me in the hall and said, 'I want to do a book for the patients.' I'd been with him long enough to know his opinion on most everything, so I drew up an outline and we got to work." That project was released in 1996 under the title *The Crystal Clear Guide to Sight for Life*, published by Starburst Publishers (Lancaster, Pa). "Some offices and ophthalmic training programs have also found that the book is an ideal guide for the beginning assistant, so its influence has gone beyond what we originally thought," she says.

During 1994 to 1996, Jan and her family moved to Aiken, SC, while her husband, Jim, attended The Medical College of Georgia. During that time, she worked for Dr. Enoch Tsai while continuing to write on the side. (Much of *The Crystal Clear Guide* was written in the parking lot of her son's elementary school in Aiken, before reporting to the office for work.) After Jim graduated, they returned to Warner Robins once again.

It was during this second stint in Warner Robins that Jan learned about SLACK's plans for the Basic Bookshelf for Eyecare Professionals, a project that was as yet unnamed and unmanned.

"I asked them who was going to be the Series' Editor, and they asked me if I'd consider it," she remembers. "It didn't take much consideration to say 'Yes!' I'd worked hard as a writer to get to that point. I was ready for something big." "Something big" is right. The Series has grown to include 25 books and has extended into a 4-year project. Would she do it again? "Yes. Absolutely. Yes." Her reply leaves no room for doubt. She wrote four of the Series books herself (the three exam review books, plus *The Slit Lamp Primer* [with Val Sanders]). She also wrote *The Complete Guide to Ocular History Taking*, which, while published by SLACK Incorporated (1999), is not part of the Series.

In the midst of her work on the Series, her family moved yet again, this time to Franklin, NC. While her ophthalmic career has taken a definite turn more toward writing and editing, she does do clinical work for Western North Carolina Eye Care Associates several days a month.

Now that she's no longer working outside the home full-time, she's had a chance to further expand as a writer. Her articles have appeared in magazines such as *The Writer, The Pen Woman, The Christian Communicator*, and the *Georgia Living and Vacation Guide*. She's had one novel published (*Hannah*, published by Guideposts Books in 1997) and is currently working on another. She's also a prize-winning short story writer, and writes a bi-weekly slice-of-life column for her hometown newspaper in Warner Robins. She is a member of the Atlanta Branch of the National League of American Pen Women, as well as two writers' groups.

She and her husband, Jim (a physician's assistant), have been married 23 years. They have two sons: TJ, a student at Western Carolina University, and Collin, a student at Franklin High School. They are all active in the First Baptist Church of Franklin, and happily share their mountain home with four cats. Jan's hobbies include singing, bowling, and reading.

Publisher's Note: The abbreviations COA, COT, COMT, and JCAHPO are registered trademarks belonging to the Joint Commission on Allied Health Personnel in Ophthalmology.

Introduction

If you've used SLACK's review books for ophthalmic assistants and technicians, you'll notice that this review book is a little bit different.

First, instead of including the chapter on how to study, we have given you hints (in the Appendix) on taking a practical exam.

Second, because of space constraints involving the title now in your hand, we were forced to limit the number of questions. (I admit, it was also to prevent me from being daunted by so large a task as trying to include every possible question!) While we have given questions and answers from each of the JCAHPO content areas for medical technologists, the material covered here is the bare basics. (The assistant and technician review books more or less covered everything. If you knew the material in those books, you would probably pass the tests. At the technologist level, however, not only is the candidate required to know material from the technologist criteria, but also material from the earlier exams *at a deeper* level.) However, I was able to "cheat" just a little by including many tables that contain information beyond what the questions ask. This way you will have material from which to study that will take you a slight step beyond the basics. You may also notice that, contrary to the other two review books, I didn't dwell so much on why the wrong answers were wrong. Instead, I tried to concentrate on making sure you had a good background in understanding what is correct. Thus, the Explanatory Answers often give more information than simply why the correct answer *is* the correct answer. When checking your responses, even if you got the answer right, it's still important that you read through the explanation. While I couldn't include all the question possibilities I would have liked to, I did try to include as much information as I could.

Also with the intention of providing a good background, in many cases the Explanatory Answers include the reference from which I got the material. That way, if there is any doubt as to the accuracy of an answer or explanation, you can go to the "horse's mouth" and see what other authors are saying. If various references provided differing information, I tell you that as well. The Bibliography at the end of the book will also provide you with much worthwhile in-depth reading as you prepare for your exam. Obviously, my major intent is to provide you with accurate information. To that end, in addition to very careful research, I also enlisted the reviewers mentioned in the Acknowledgments. However, if you find a problem with the answer to any question, please contact me through the Publisher. We are constantly striving to make these review books accurate and useful, and we depend on the assistance of the readers to achieve those goals.

Along the same line, we would also appreciate hearing from you after you take the exam. Your comments on the appropriateness of the review questions will be seriously considered. In addition, you might let us know which sections were most helpful.

Students often want to know what reference material will be the most essential as they prepare for an exam. My reference list for this review book is lengthy; it would be very difficult, even if you had access to the same material, for you to study it all. But assuming that you already have a basic text or two on ophthalmology and/or ophthalmic assisting (notably, something like *General Ophthalmology* by Vaughan, Asbury, and Riordan-Eva, published by Appleton and Lange), here are my two favorite references that should go a long way in getting you prepared: *Special Skills and Techniques*, by Gretchen Van Boemel (SLACK Incorporated) and *Manual of Ocular Diagnosis and Therapy*, edited by Deborah Pavan-Langston (Little, Brown, and Co).

Also useful at this level are the Basic Bookshelf books: *Clinical Ocular Photography; Optics, Retinoscopy, and Refractometry; Ophthalmic Medications and Pharmacology; A Systematic*

Approach to Strabismus; and *Visual Fields*. Access to a set of *Duane's Ophthalmology* (on CD-ROM is best, by Lippincott-Raven Publishers) is good, too.

Because the Joint Commission is constantly reviewing the content areas to make sure that they are appropriate for the needs of physicians (and patients) as well as expanding technology, it's vital that you have the most current copy of the exam criteria. This can be obtained by contacting JCAHPO at 1-800-284-3937 or e-mailing them at jcahpo@jcahpo.org. Their Internet address is http://www.jcahpo.org.

Chapter 1

Microbiology

1. **The four classic signs of inflammation are:**
   a) itching, swelling, redness, and discharge
   b) redness, swelling, warmth, and pain
   c) redness, discharge, fever, and pain
   d) tingling, rash, fever, and discharge

2. **Two of the chemical mediators of the inflammatory response are:**
   a) histamine and prostaglandins
   b) epinephrine and norepinephrine
   c) estrogen and progesterone
   d) insulin and glucogen

3. **The formation of antibodies by the host is stimulated by the presence of a(n):**
   a) inoculation
   b) antigen
   c) histamine
   d) fever

4. **The substance that binds to an antibody and results in the destruction of the cell is:**
   a) hormone
   b) synapse
   c) antigen
   d) complement

5. **Infectious agents that can cause an inflammatory response in the eye include:**
   a) *Pseudomonas aeruginosa*, *Herpes*, and *Chlamydia*
   b) *Candida albicans*, *Toxocara canis*, and *Acanthameobae*
   c) bacteria, viruses, and fungi
   d) all of the above

6. **As related to toxicity, a highly aggressive pathogen would be described as:**
   a) deadly
   b) barely virulent
   c) moderately virulent
   d) highly virulent

7. **A pathogen can cause an inflammatory reaction due to:**
   a) production of toxins and/or enzymes
   b) reproduction within the host's cells
   c) an allergic reaction to toxins
   d) all of the above

8. **Examples of non-infectious causes of the inflammatory response are:**
   a) trauma, inheritance, autoimmunity, and nutritional
   b) bacterial, viral, and fungal
   c) hormonal, growth, and developmental
   d) digestive, respiratory, and cardiovascular

9. **Papillae, infiltrates, hypopyon, and exudates are all manifestations of:**
    a) inflammatory cells
    b) hereditary disorders
    c) hormonal reactions
    d) blood-borne pathogens

10. **Neutrophils, eosinophils, and basophils are all types of:**
    a) lymphocytes
    b) red blood cells
    c) antibodies
    d) granulocytes

11. **Which of the following inflammatory cell types is most associated with allergic inflammation?**
    a) lymphocytes
    b) eosinophils
    c) neutrophils
    d) basophils

12. **These cells have a dark blue nucleus and are the chief cell seen in chronic inflammation:**
    a) lymphocytes
    b) neutrophils
    c) eosinophils
    d) hemoglobes

13. **Histamine is released from this inflammatory cell:**
    a) basophile (mast cell)
    b) neutrophile
    c) eosinophile
    d) plasma cell

14. **Antibodies are produced by these cells that have a dark blue eccentric nucleus:**
    a) granulocyte
    b) plasma cell
    c) red blood cell
    d) neutrophile

15. **The monocyte (macrophage or histiocyte):**
    a) has a round nucleus and is the major phagocytic cell type
    b) has no nucleus and is the major phagocytic cell type
    c) has an oval or horseshoe-shaped blue nucleus and releases histamine
    d) has an oval or horseshoe-shaped blue nucleus and is the major phagocytic cell type

16. **An inflammatory cell with a multi-lobed nucleus that might be seen in a staphylococcal infection is:**
    a) neutrophile (polymorphonucleocyte or PMN)
    b) macrophage
    c) red blood cell
    d) basophile

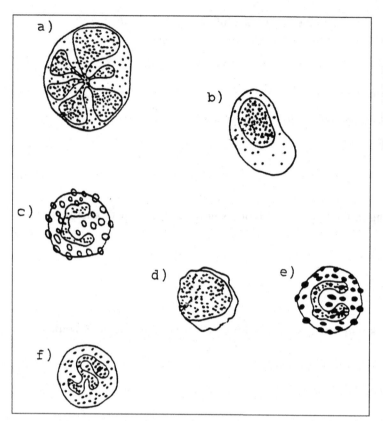

Figure 1-1. Inflammatory cells. (Composed of drawings from Nemeth SC, Shea CA. *Medical Sciences for the Ophthalmic Assistant.* Thorofare, NJ: SLACK Incorporated; 1988. Reprinted with permission.)

17 through 22. Identify the inflammatory cell types represented in Figure 1-1:
basophile (mast cell)
plasma cell
eosinophile
monocyte (macrophage/histiocyte)
lymphocyte
neutrophile (PMN)

23. Bacteria may be identified based on:
a) whether or not the disorder is fatal
b) shape, staining characteristics, and culture characteristics
c) mortality, epidemiology, and microbiology
d) disorder characteristics, morbidity, and species

24. Round bacteria that appear singly, paired, clustered, or chained are:
a) bacilli
b) spirochetes
c) diplo
d) cocci

25. *Pseudomonas aeruginosa, Haemophilus influenzae,* and *Mycobacterium tuberculosis* all fall into the category of:
    a) rod-shaped bacilli
    b) sickle-shaped bacilli
    c) round diplococci
    d) clustered cocci

26. An example of a spirochete (spiral-shaped bacteria) is:
    a) *Staphylococcus aureus*
    b) *Streptococcus pneumonia*
    c) *Treponema pallidum*
    d) *Herpes zoster*

27. You are examining a smear from a patient with a corneal ulcer. The slide was prepared with Giemsa stain, and you can see extra, stained structures in the cells. These are most likely:
    a) viral spores
    b) inclusion bodies
    c) fungal spores
    d) Giemsa stain is not used for this purpose

28. You are examining a smear from a patient with chronic blepharitis. You see round gram-positive bacteria arranged in clusters. Most likely, the infection is due to:
    a) *Streptococcus*
    b) *Haemophilus influenzae*
    c) *Pseudomonas aeruginosa*
    d) *Staphylococcus*

29. Your patient has cellulitis with a history of penetrating injury to the lids. You find gram-positive cocci arranged in chains. This indicates that the infection is probably due to:
    a) *Treponema pallidum*
    b) *Chlamydia*
    c) *Staphylococcus*
    d) *Streptococcus*

30. Your patient has ulcerative blepharoconjunctivitis, which the physician suspects is due to second-stage syphilis. When examining a smear from this patient under the microscope, you would expect to find:
    a) gram-positive cocci arranged in chains
    b) a slender gram-negative spirochete with a flagellum, using dark-field illumination
    c) a slender gram-positive spirochete with a flagellum, using dark-field illumination
    d) gram-negative sickle-shaped cells

31. The bacterium implicated in Question 30 is:
    a) *Treponema pallidum*
    b) *Staphylococcus aureus*
    c) *Haemophilus*
    d) *Neisseria gonorrhoea*

32. A patient with conjunctivitis gives a history of pneumonia. If the infection is due to *Strep pneumonia*, you will examine the smear for:
    a) gram-positive tiny, slender rods in chains
    b) gram-positive diplococci that are lancet shaped
    c) gram-positive cocci that cluster in a lancet shape
    d) gram-negative kidney-shaped cells that are paired

33. You are asked to examine a smear taken from an infant with severe conjunctivitis. If the patient has ophthalmia neonatorum caused by *Neisseria gonorrhoea*, you would expect to see:
    a) gram-negative bacteria that are paired and kidney-shaped
    b) gram-negative bacteria that have flagella
    c) gram-positive cocci in clusters
    d) virus particles

34. The classification of bacteria according to their staining properties is dependent on the bacterium's:
    a) envelope
    b) nucleus
    c) cytoplasm
    d) mitochondria

35. The three main groupings of bacteria according to staining properties are:
    a) gram-positive, gram-negative, and acid-fast
    b) gram-positive, gram-negative, and dark-field illumination
    c) Wright-positive, Wright-negative, and Gram-fast
    d) gram-positive, gram-negative, and Giemsa-fast

36. The classic stain that helps identify bacteria according to whether or not it is absorbed by the cell wall is:
    a) India ink
    b) Giemsa stain
    c) Gram stain
    d) Wright stain

37. If the stain mentioned in Question 36 is not absorbed by the bacterial cell wall, that organism is classified as:
    a) Wright-negative
    b) acid-fast
    c) gram-positive
    d) gram-negative

38. You have performed a Gram stain on a conjunctival smear. Under the microscope, you observe red, round bacteria. This organism is:
    a) gram-negative
    b) gram-positive
    c) Giemsa-positive
    d) acid-fast

39. **You are evaluating a smear taken from an hypopyon. If the cause of the infection is *Candida albicans* and the stain has been prepared with Gram stain, you will see:**
    a) green-stained organisms
    b) black, counterstained organisms
    c) reddish pink-stained organisms
    d) dark blue-stained organisms

40. **If one suspected a chlamydial infection, the smear should be stained with:**
    a) Gram stain
    b) acid-fast stain
    c) Giemsa stain
    d) India ink

41. **In order to identify inflammatory cells, a smear should be stained with:**
    a) Giemsa or Wright stain
    b) Gram stain or India ink
    c) Gram or acid-fast stain
    d) Giemsa or Gram stain

42. **A patient has a corneal ulcer. In order to rule out a fungal origin, you should stain the smear with:**
    a) India ink
    b) Giemsa stain
    c) acid-fast stain
    d) methylene blue

43. **If a bacteria's capsule is resistant to staining, a negative stain may be used so that the organism will show up against a darkly stained background. One stain used for this purpose is:**
    a) methylene blue
    b) Wright stain
    c) India ink
    d) Giemsa stain

44. **One bacterium that might be stained negatively in order to aid in its identification is**
    a) *Streptococcus pneumoniae*
    b) *Staphylococcus aureus*
    c) *Haemophilus*
    d) *Candida*

45. ***Mycobacterium tuberculosis* is traditionally stained with:**
    a) India ink
    b) acid-fast stain
    c) Gram stain
    d) methylene blue

46. **Various types of media include:**
    a) dyes, stains, and cultures
    b) ices, broths, and gels
    c) agar plate, agar slant, and broth
    d) swabs, spatulas, and loops

47. **In order to support the growth of specific organisms:**
    a) carbon dioxide must always be provided
    b) nutrients such as blood or dextrose may be added to the medium
    c) dyes are added to the medium
    d) the inoculated plate may be coated with dextrose

48. **If blood agar is heated, this produces:**
    a) chocolate agar
    b) chocolate broth
    c) agar coagulase
    d) Sabouraud agar

49. **An infant is suspected to have neonatal conjunctivitis due to *Neisseria gonorrhoeae*. The medium of choice is:**
    a) Thayer Martin agar plate
    b) Sabouraud agar
    c) plain agar
    d) Thioglycolate broth

50. **In order to culture fungi, the medium of choice would be:**
    a) blood agar
    b) chocolate agar
    c) Thioglycolate broth
    d) Sabouraud dextrose agar

51. **An antibiotic may be added to fungal culture medium in order to:**
    a) retard the growth of bacteria in the culture
    b) encourage the growth of symbiotic bacteria
    c) increase fungal growth rate
    d) prevent infection to lab personnel

52. **Placing antibiotic disks on an inoculated culture helps identify:**
    a) which antibiotic to give the patient
    b) how to kill the culture
    c) the difference between gram-positive and gram-negative bacteria
    d) what vaccine to give the patient

53. **In which of the following cases might a culture be ordered?**
    a) chronic conjunctivitis
    b) orbital cellulitis
    c) postoperative infections
    d) all of the above

54. **Which of the following would be used to culture a virus?**
    a) blood agar
    b) chocolate agar
    c) tissue cultures and chick embryo membranes
    d) only broths may be used

55. **Of the following, which would be most difficult to culture?**
    a) *Mulluscum contagiosum*
    b) *Neisseria gonorrhoea*
    c) *Staphylococcus*
    d) *Streptococcus*

56. **When obtaining material for a conjunctival culture it is important to:**
    a) use topical anesthesia before taking the smear
    b) avoid any discharge that is present
    c) swab both the conjunctiva and lid margin
    d) use a sterile swab moistened with sterile saline solution

57. **A corneal scraping might be indicated in cases of:**
    a) corneal ulcer
    b) corneal dystrophy
    c) contact lens over-wear
    d) corneal abrasion of unknown origin

58. **When taking a corneal scraping, it is important to:**
    a) use a topical anesthetic prior to the scraping
    b) apply the spatula while it is hot
    c) obtain material from the center of the ulcer
    d) rub the spatula back and forth across the ulcer

59. **When obtaining material from the lid margin for a culture or smear, one should first:**
    a) cleanse the area with iodine
    b) remove crusts and scales from the lid margin
    c) trim the lashes to avoid contamination
    d) apply antibacterial ointment

60. **In addition to traditional lid margin, conjunctival, and corneal smears, material may be taken for smears or cultures from:**
    a) the anterior chamber via a tap
    b) any excised tissue
    c) the meibomian glands, canaliculi, and lacrimal sac
    d) all of the above

61. **In order to comply with health and safety guidelines, one should:**
    a) wear gloves when taking a culture or scraping
    b) dispose of contaminated materials in a biohazard waste receptacle
    c) fix the smear or inoculate the culture immediately
    d) all of the above

62. **In addition to identifying a specimen by patient name and number, it is also important to note:**
    a) the date and origin of the material
    b) the suspected organism
    c) the patient's treatment regimen
    d) the temperature of the room where the specimen was taken

63. **Identifying the eye from which a culture is taken may be done by:**
    a) tracing an L or an R on the agar during inoculation
    b) inverting the plate if from the right eye, not inverting the plate if from the left eye
    c) placing a paper tag on the agar surface
    d) placing a label on the inside of the dish top

64. **When smearing material on a microscope slide for examination, one should:**
    a) spread the material as thinly as possible
    b) spread the material across the entire slide surface
    c) arrange the material in a clump, then press it down with a cover slip
    d) allow the slide to air dry first

65. **"Fixing" a smear on a microscope slide refers to the process of:**
    a) rapidly hardening and preserving tissue elements
    b) holding it under rapidly running hot water to remove contaminants
    c) gluing a cover slip over the smear
    d) applying stain to the smear

66. **Methods of fixing a smear include:**
    a) air drying
    b) flame drying
    c) chemicals
    d) all of the above

67. **You wish to use Gram stain on a slide. You should fix the material by:**
    a) allowing it to air dry
    b) rinsing it with alcohol
    c) blowing on it
    d) gentle flaming

68. **In addition to Gram's iodine, these solutions are necessary to make a Gram stain:**
    a) India ink, denatured water, acetone, and safranin
    b) methanol, gentian violet, basic salt solution, and acetone
    c) gentian violet, tap water, ethyl alcohol or acetone, and safranin
    d) methanol, tap water, methylene blue, and fuchsin solution

69. **The proper sequence for making a Gram stain is:**
    a) fixation, crystal violet, water rinse, Gram's iodine, water rinse, ethyl alcohol or acetone, water rinse, safranin, water rinse, blot dry
    b) fixation, Gram's iodine, water rinse, crystal violet, acetone rinse, water rinse, flame dry
    c) fixation, Gram's iodine, water rinse, India ink, water rinse, acetone, water rinse, safranin, air dry
    d) fixation, Gram's iodine, methanol rinse, methylene blue, water rinse, fuchsin solution, water rinse, blot dry

70. **When performing a Gram stain, the gentian violet and Gram's iodine should be used:**
    a) for equal amounts of time
    b) for 5 minutes each
    c) in a double-dilution formula
    d) in a 2:1 ratio

71. **During Gram staining, when flooding the slide with ethyl alcohol or acetone, one must be careful:**
    a) not to over-stain
    b) not to apply it for less than 30 seconds
    c) to flame the slide immediately afterwards
    d) not to over-decolorize

72. **The purpose of the safranin used in the Gram staining process is:**
    a) as a counterstain to make the gram-negative organisms visible
    b) as a counterstain to make the gram-positive organisms visible
    c) to decolorize
    d) as a "glue" to hold on the cover slip

73. **If one needed a cell-differentiating stain in a hurry, the stain of choice would be:**
    a) Giemsa stain
    b) Wright stain
    c) methylene blue stain
    d) India ink stain

74. **The proper dilution for Giemsa stain is:**
    a) 2 parts stain to 1 part distilled water
    b) 2 mL of stain in 50 mL acetone
    c) 2 mL of Giemsa in 50 mL distilled water
    d) in equal amounts

75. **Once the slide is fixed, the properly diluted Giemsa stain is allowed to:**
    a) totally cover the slide for 40 to 60 minutes
    b) contact the slide for only 1 to 2 seconds
    c) constantly trickle over the slide for 5 minutes
    d) cover the slide for 10 to 15 minutes

76. **After the slide has been in the Giemsa stain for the required time, the next step is to:**
    a) flame the slide
    b) immerse in tap water for 5 minutes
    c) rinse with distilled water until clear
    d) rinse briefly with ethyl alcohol two times

77. **For a Wright stain, the stain is applied to the smear and allowed to remain for:**
    a) 1 minute
    b) 5 minutes
    c) 20 minutes
    d) 40 to 60 minutes

78. **After staining, the next step for a Wright stain is to:**
    a) pour off the stain and rinse
    b) rinse with methanol
    c) add water to the stain for 10 minutes
    d) flood the slide with safranin

79. **The final step in making a Wright stain is to:**
    a) rinse with water and air dry
    b) rinse with acetone and air dry
    c) rinse with water and flame dry
    d) rinse with methanol and flame dry

80. **When inoculating an agar plate, one should:**
    a) gently streak the swab in lines over the agar surface
    b) stab the agar surface with the cotton swab
    c) use a gloved finger to gently spread the smear evenly over the agar surface
    d) gently rub the swab over the entire agar surface

81. **When placing an agar plate into the incubator, one should:**
    a) stack the plates sideways
    b) remove the plate cover
    c) invert the plate (agar side up)
    d) place the plate agar side down

82. **If a test tube of broth is used as a medium, one may obtain the swab with a cotton-tipped applicator. The applicator is then:**
    a) broken off and left in the broth
    b) flamed to sterilize it
    c) reapplied to the eye to obtain another sample
    d) squeezed to remove all traces of the broth

83. **Most bacterial cultures are incubated at:**
    a) 35 to 37 degrees C
    b) 25 degrees C
    c) 15 to 20 degrees C
    d) 0 degrees C

84. **If there is little or no bacterial growth on a plate in the first 24 hours of incubation:**
    a) the culture is incubated for another 24 hours
    b) a "no growth" report is sent and the plate discarded
    c) a repeat culture is taken
    d) a different medium should be tried

85. **When evaluating cultured bacterial colonies, one should note:**
    a) size, shape, and color
    b) number of colonies
    c) odor and media changes
    d) all of the above

86. **A common fungal contaminant that often grows in bacterial cultures is:**
    a) *Aspergillus*
    b) *Chlamydia*
    c) *Candida*
    d) *Acanthomeobae*

87. **The rate of growth in a fungal culture:**
    a) is more rapid than bacteria
    b) is enhanced by increased moisture and cooler temperatures
    c) is about the same as that of bacteria
    d) is slow

88. **Viral and *Chlamydia* cultures are prepared for transfer to a virology lab by using:**
    a) wet ice (4 degrees C)
    b) dry ice (carbon dioxide snow)
    c) a heat pack to maintain 98.6 degrees F
    d) a chemical pack to maintain carbon dioxide levels

Chapter 2

Advanced Tonometry

1. **The theory of nerve death (caused by glaucoma) that states that the axons die due to inadequate blood flow is the:**
   a) indirect mechanical theory
   b) direct ischemic theory
   c) direct mechanical theory
   d) indirect ischemic theory

2. **The theory of nerve fiber damage (caused by glaucoma) that states that the axons die due to compression of the nerve fibers is the:**
   a) direct ischemic theory
   b) direct mechanical theory
   c) indirect mechanical theory
   d) indirect ischemic theory

3. **Elevated intraocular pressure (IOP) as seen in chronic open-angle glaucoma is believed to be the result of:**
   a) decreased function and/or density of cells in the trabecular meshwork
   b) obstruction of the trabecular meshwork by particulate matter
   c) overproduction of aqueous
   d) optic nerve damage

4. **Chronic glaucoma causes atrophy of the pars plicata and fibrosis of the ciliary processes, evidence of damage to the:**
   a) optic nerve
   b) cup-to-disc ratio
   c) ganglion cells
   d) ciliary body

5. **In an adult, if IOP is elevated over a long period of time (as in chronic glaucoma), the following change may be seen:**
   a) enlarged cornea
   b) buphthalmos
   c) scleral thinning
   d) ciliary flush

6. **The retinal damage of chronic glaucoma is manifested by damage to:**
   a) the nerve fiber and ganglion cell layers
   b) the macula
   c) the retinal vascular system
   d) the photoreceptor cells

7. **The focal point of optic nerve damage in glaucoma is the:**
   a) lamina cribrosa
   b) myelin sheath
   c) hyaloid membrane
   d) embryonic layer

8. **The type of early glaucoma field loss that occurs most often is:**
   a) nasal steps
   b) temporal wedges
   c) paracentral scotomas in the Bjerrum area
   d) concentric contraction

9. **A poorer prognosis exists for the patient who has:**
   a) enlarged blind spots
   b) nasal steps
   c) Seidel scotoma in the superior field
   d) Bjerrum scotoma in the superior field and Seidel scotoma in the inferior field

10. **Visual acuity in a glaucoma patient with a 10 degree island of central vision and a detached, large temporal island (in the absence of other ocular disease) might be expected to be:**
    a) 20/20
    b) 20/100
    c) 20/200
    d) less than 20/400

11. **The patient described in Question 10 would most likely find which activity difficult?**
    a) reading
    b) watching TV
    c) driving
    d) sewing

12. **Once the patient has only a temporal island of vision remaining, the IOP should be kept very low because of:**
    a) the snuff-out phenomenon
    b) pressure spikes
    c) restricted visual fields
    d) decreased efficacy of medications

13. **It is thought by some investigators that, preceding changes in the visual field, the glaucoma patient might exhibit changes in:**
    a) color vision and contrast sensitivity
    b) central vision
    c) Amsler grid testing
    d) stereopsis and motility function

14. **Unstable thresholds, transient areas of field loss, and shallow defects may be associated with:**
    a) end-stage glaucoma field loss
    b) tunnel vision
    c) moderate glaucoma field loss
    d) early or impending glaucoma field loss

15. **Secondary glaucoma can be classified as:**
    a) absolute or partial
    b) hypotony or supraelevation
    c) pre-trabecular, trabecular, or post-trabecular
    d) medical or non-medical

16. **Treatment of secondary glaucoma primarily consists of:**
    a) laser surgery
    b) beta blockers
    c) miotics to prevent angle closure
    d) finding the root cause and treating that

17. **A hypermature cataract may cause secondary glaucoma by:**
    a) leaking proteins that clog the trabeculum
    b) dislocating and drifting into the anterior chamber
    c) dislocating and drifting into the vitreous
    d) exfoliating

18. **Neovascular glaucoma would most likely be seen in a patient with:**
    a) diabetes
    b) contact lens over-wear
    c) high blood pressure
    d) carotid artery disease

19. **Patients who experience an increase in IOP while using corticosteroids are called:**
    a) ocular hypertensives
    b) glaucoma suspects
    c) steroid regulators
    d) steroid responders

20. **Patients with asthma, emphysema, and renal transplants should have their IOP monitored regularly because:**
    a) patients with these disorders commonly take steroids
    b) they tend to develop vascular glaucoma
    c) they tend to develop malignant glaucoma
    d) these conditions predispose one to angle closure

21. **Malignant glaucoma is a postoperative complication that occurs when:**
    a) aqueous leaks into the vitreous
    b) vitreous strands are present in the anterior chamber
    c) conjunctival epithelium invades the angle structures
    d) there is a hemorrhage in the anterior chamber

22. **Slit lamp signs that often accompany pigmentary glaucoma include:**
    a) Vossius ring
    b) crocodile shagreen
    c) Krukenberg's spindles and iris transillumination defects
    d) iron pigment line and arcus senilus

23. **Physicians do not rely on IOP measurements alone when evaluating a patient for glaucoma because:**
    a) some eyes cannot tolerate even "normal" pressure
    b) tonometers are difficult to calibrate
    c) only Goldmann tonometry is reliable
    d) inaccuracies are common

24. **Ocular hypertension is a situation in which there is elevated IOP:**
    a) but the cup-to-disc ratio is less than 0.4
    b) but no damage has occurred to the optic nerve or visual field
    c) and nerve damage has remained stable over a period of years
    d) and the patient also has high blood pressure

25. **A patient who is a "glaucoma suspect" is:**
    a) at risk for developing glaucoma
    b) a candidate for immediate endolaser treatment
    c) a candidate for preventative laser iridotomies
    d) 100% sure of developing glaucoma eventually

26. **Congenital glaucoma in which the trabeculum and Schlemm's canal did not develop normally is a type of:**
    a) acquired congenital glaucoma
    b) secondary congenital glaucoma
    c) isolated congenital glaucoma
    d) all of the above

27. **Symptoms of congenital glaucoma may include:**
    a) redness and decreased vision
    b) swelling, photophobia, and diplopia
    c) epiphora, redness, and mattering
    d) photophobia, blepharospasm, and epiphora

28. **Because an infant's sclera is more elastic than an adult's, elevated IOP may cause:**
    a) buphthalmos
    b) blanched sclera
    c) yellow sclera
    d) scleral show

29. **Corneal enlargement may occur due to elevated IOP. An infant's corneal diameter is considered abnormal (and suspicious for congenital glaucoma) if it is:**
    a) larger than 10.5 mm
    b) larger than 10.0 mm
    c) larger than 9.5 mm
    d) larger than 9.0 mm

30. **When IOP is measured in a newborn, the patient is suspicious for congenital glaucoma if the reading is:**
    a) higher than 12 mmHg
    b) higher than 18 mmHg
    c) higher than 22 mmHg
    d) higher than 26 mmHg

31. **Treatment of choice for isolated congenital glaucoma is:**
    a) goniotomy or trabeculotomy
    b) beta blockers
    c) carbonic anhydrase inhibitors
    d) laser iridotomy

32. **A tonometer that, when applied to the eye, raises the IOP only by a negligible amount is known as a:**
    a) Goldmann tonometer
    b) low-displacement tonometer
    c) Schiotz tonometer
    d) high-displacement tonometer

33. **The principle that states that the pressure inside a sphere can be measured by applying an equal amount of pressure on the outside of the sphere is:**
    a) Imbert-Fick
    b) Mackay-Marg
    c) Roadarmel-Ledford
    d) Friedenwald

34. **The Goldmann and Mackay-Marg tonometers are examples of:**
    a) fixed area tonometers
    b) fixed force tonometers
    c) fixed optical tonometers
    d) fixed mires tonometers

35. **The non-contact "air-puff" tonometer is an example of:**
    a) applanation tonometry
    b) indentation tonometry
    c) fixed force tonometry
    d) manometry

36. **With the Goldmann applanation tonometer, how much aqueous is displaced during the measurement?**
    a) 0.5 microliters
    b) 5.0 microliters
    c) 0.1 microliters
    d) 0.05 microliters

37. **The principle that a gas- or fluid-filled sphere will be indented *more* by a given weight if the sphere's internal pressure is low (vs being indented less if the internal pressure is high) is the basis for:**
    a) indentation tonometry
    b) applanation tonometry
    c) fixed area tonometry
    d) manometry

38. **With the Schiotz tonometer, the scale moves up 1 unit for each:**
    a) 1.0 mm that the plunger falls below the footplate
    b) 0.5 mm that the plunger falls below the footplate
    c) 0.1 mm that the plunger falls below the footplate
    d) 0.05 mm that the plunger falls below the footplate

39. **The relationship between the amount of indentation (with the Schiotz tonometer) and the IOP:**
    a) is inversely proportional
    b) is logarithmic
    c) is linear
    d) is geometric

40. **If the same eye was measured with the Schiotz tonometer using each of the tonometer weights (supposing that, in this case, repeated measurements would not force aqueous from the chamber), one would find:**
    a) the patient's diurnal curve
    b) the same IOP measurement
    c) progressively higher IOP measurements
    d) progressively lower IOP measurements

41. **All of the following are true about the Schiotz conversion tables *except*:**
    a) it is based on cadaver eyes
    b) it is based on normal scleral rigidity
    c) each table is specific to that instrument
    d) it was developed by Friedenwald

42. **Using the Goldmann tonometer on an edematous or scarred cornea will generally cause measurements that are:**
    a) higher than the actual IOP
    b) lower than the actual IOP
    c) reliable enough to be accepted
    d) unreliable because fluorescein cannot be used

43. **Measuring a scarred cornea with the Schiotz tonometer will be inaccurate because:**
    a) the weight will distort the cornea
    b) the gauge will pulsate
    c) the mires will be distorted
    d) the eye will tend to have a high scleral rigidity

44. **A scarred, irregular cornea is difficult to measure with the Goldmann tonometer because:**
    a) there is decreased scleral rigidity
    b) one cannot instill topical anesthetic because of tissue melt
    c) one cannot use fluorescein because it will infiltrate the tissue
    d) the mires are irregular, making it difficult to judge the endpoint

45. **The tonometer of choice when measuring IOP in a patient who has had a recent corneal graft is the:**
    a) Schiotz
    b) Goldmann
    c) non-contact
    d) Mackay-Marg

46. **In the presence of a diseased, irregular cornea, the Mackay-Marg or Tono-Pen are advantageous because:**
    a) topical anesthetic is not required
    b) no fluorescein is required
    c) the mires are more clear
    d) the IOP can be measured through a bandage contact lens

47. **If the cornea is extremely thick or scarred:**
    a) the IOP measurements will always be underestimated
    b) the IOP measurements will always be overestimated
    c) the IOP measurements can be accepted with reservations
    d) no tonometric measurement will be accurate enough to satisfy clinical needs

48. **One must make an adjustment to the Goldmann or Perkins tonoprism if the patient's corneal astigmatism is:**
    a) greater than 1 D
    b) greater than 2 D
    c) greater than 3 D
    d) greater than 4 D

49. **If compensation for high corneal astigmatism is not made (to the Goldmann or Perkins tonometers), the IOP measurement could be in error by:**
    a) 1 mmHg
    b) 2 to 3 mmHg
    c) 4 to 5 mmHg
    d) 8 to 10 mmHg

50. **In order to compensate for high astigmatism with the Goldmann or Perkins tonometers, the biprism should be aligned as follows:**
    a) the steepest axis aligned with the red line
    b) the plus axis aligned with the red line
    c) 45 degrees from the minus cylinder should be placed in the 90 degree position
    d) the minus axis aligned with the red line

Chapter 3

Advanced
Visual Fields

1. **In kinetic perimetry, the target is moved from non-seeing to seeing at a rate of:**
   a) 1 to 2 degrees per second
   b) 2 to 3 degrees per second
   c) 4 to 5 degrees per minute
   d) 4 to 5 degrees per second

2. **With kinetic perimetry, except for any physiologic blind spots, it is assumed that:**
   a) the examiner's visual field is normal
   b) all areas inside the isopter will respond to the same stimulus
   c) all areas outside the isopter will respond to the same stimulus
   d) all areas outside the isopter will respond to a dimmer stimulus

3. **When testing the visual field with kinetic techniques, an abnormality will be illustrated by:**
   a) a single spot where the stimulus is not seen
   b) a displacement in the usual position of the isopter boundary
   c) an area where the isopter boundary is expanded
   d) a single spot where a dimmer stimulus is not seen

4. **The Armaly-Drance method of visual field screening for glaucoma consists of:**
   a) kinetic methods
   b) static methods
   c) both kinetic and static methods
   d) automated fields only

5. **Automated static perimetry is considered more accurate for the glaucoma field because:**
   a) it takes less time
   b) it is easier to detect defects in Bjerrum's area
   c) it is a more sensitive test
   d) all of the above

6. **Measurements using static threshold perimetry with the Goldmann perimeter are made:**
   a) every 3 to 5 degrees along a single meridian
   b) every 1 to 2 degrees along a single meridian
   c) every 5 to 10 degrees along a single meridian
   d) every 10 to 12 degrees along the horizontal meridian only

7. **After the appropriate adjustment in stimulus intensity following a patient's response at a given point during a static test, the patient changes the response the next time the point is tested (ie, seen one time and not seen the next, or vice versa). Threshold has thus been:**
   a) exhausted
   b) staircased
   c) crossed
   d) bracketed

8. **Binocular field testing is used primarily in patients who have:**
   a) glaucoma
   b) restrictive or paralytic strabismus
   c) amblyopia
   d) phorias

9. **Which of the following is best for binocular field testing?**
   a) automated perimeter
   b) Goldmann perimeter
   c) tangent screen
   d) confrontation fields

10. **Which of the following is *not* true regarding binocular field testing?**
    a) neither eye is occluded
    b) corrective lenses are used as in regular field testing
    c) the patient is told to hold fixation on the central target
    d) if the patient reports that the stimulus is doubled, the target is moved slowly until he or she states it is single

11. **The appropriate target in binocular field testing is:**
    a) red or green
    b) at threshold for the central 30
    c) at threshold for the periphery
    d) one that is easily seen

12. **The results of a binocular field are generally not a consideration in disability if diplopia occurs:**
    a) within the central 30 degrees
    b) outside the central 20 degrees
    c) outside the central 30 degrees
    d) in the inferior meridians

13. **What type of defect is most commonly seen when optic nerve damage is due to toxicity?**
    a) nasal step
    b) paracentral/centrocecal scotoma
    c) "pie in the sky"
    d) "pie on the floor"

14. **Which of the following is generally affected by toxicity from lead poisoning and methyl alcohol?**
    a) the papillomacular bundle
    b) the macula
    c) the optic nerve
    d) all of the above

15. **The visual field defect seen in tobacco-alcohol amblyopia is:**
    a) nasal step
    b) enlarged blind spot
    c) tubular fields
    d) centrocecal scotoma

16. **In general, if one detects a visual field defect that is suspicious for toxicity, which of the following will generally be present as well?**
    a) decreased visual acuity and color vision
    b) floaters and flashes
    c) a decrease in media clarity
    d) elevated IOP

17. **A sloping isopter or scotoma margin indicates:**
    a) that sensitivity decreases gradually
    b) that sensitivity decreases suddenly
    c) that sensitivity is normal
    d) that sensitivity cannot be accurately mapped

18. **When mapping isopters with consecutively brighter stimuli, if the margins are steep, one will note:**
    a) that the isopter boundaries are equidistant from one another
    b) that the isopter boundaries are spaced farther and farther apart
    c) that the isopter boundaries are extremely close and may even be superimposed
    d) scotomata between the isopters

19. **The normal field of vision is steeper:**
    a) on the nasal side
    b) on the temporal side
    c) the farther away you get from fixation
    d) if the patient's vision is 20/40 or better

20. **A visual field defect caused by a progressive tumor would most likely exhibit:**
    a) a sudden drop-off
    b) gradually sloping margins
    c) tightly grouped isopter boundaries
    d) nasal steps

21. **An absolute scotoma responds to:**
    a) a dimmer intensity than on the last testing
    b) the minimum intensity available on that perimeter
    c) no stimulus whatsoever
    d) no stimulus available on that perimeter, including the brightest

22. **If a patient responds only to a stimulus projected within a scotoma that is larger or brighter than the isopter's target, this is termed:**
    a) a relative scotoma
    b) an absolute scotoma
    c) a positive scotoma
    d) a negative scotoma

23. **Which of the following would be most likely to appear as an absolute scotoma?**
    a) angiod streak
    b) retinal hole
    c) drusen
    d) choroidal nevus

24. **A nasal step often begins as a(n):**
    a) arcuate scotoma
    b) nasal notch
    c) enlarged blind spot
    d) Bjerrum's scotoma

25. **The configuration of nasal step defects occurs because:**
    a) the nerve fibers do not cross the horizontal raphe
    b) the nerve fibers do not cross the vertical raphe
    c) the nose obstructs the nasal visual field
    d) the retinal tissue is tightly adherent at the 180 degree demarcation

26. **In the absence of other findings (such as a paracentral scotoma), the definition of a nasal step is:**
    a) a 5 degree difference between the superior and inferior isopters
    b) a 15 degree difference between the superior and inferior isopters
    c) a 20 degree difference between the superior and inferior isopters
    d) a 10 degree difference between the superior and inferior isopters

27. **The most common cause of a nasal step defect is:**
    a) glaucoma
    b) retinal detachment
    c) thyroid dysfunction
    d) artifact

28. **Important features of scotomata include:**
    a) density
    b) size and shape
    c) position
    d) all of the above

29. **The most common type of scotoma that occurs with optic nerve damage is the:**
    a) central scotoma
    b) junctional scotoma
    c) ring scotoma
    d) negative scotoma

30. **Unilateral scotomata generally occur:**
    a) in the retina, optic nerve, or nerve fiber layer
    b) at the chiasm
    c) in the optic radiations
    d) in the occipital lobe

31. **A junctional scotoma might be seen in a patient with:**
    a) glaucoma
    b) macular hole
    c) a pituitary tumor
    d) retinitis pigmentosa

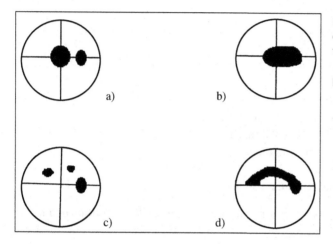

Figure 3-1. Monocular visual field defects. (Reprinted with permission from Choplin N, Edwards R. *Visual Fields.* Thorofare, NJ: SLACK Incorporated; 1998.)

32. **Label the following scotomata (Figure 3-1):**
    paracentral scotoma
    central scotoma
    arcuate scotoma
    centrocecal scotoma

33. **The condition that most often causes enlargement of the blind spot is:**
    a) papilledema
    b) glaucoma
    c) uveitis
    d) pituitary tumor

34. **An altitudinal defect usually occurs:**
    a) pre-chiasmally
    b) at the chiasm
    c) in the optic radiations
    d) in the occipital lobe

35. **A common cause of a defect in the superior field is:**
    a) superior retinal detachment
    b) ptosis
    c) pituitary tumor
    d) cataract

36. **"Pie in the sky" and "pie on the floor" altitudinal defects occur:**
    a) in the retina
    b) in the optic nerve
    c) at the chiasm
    d) in the optic radiations

Chapter 4

Advanced Color Vision

1. **Normal color vision is referred to as trichromatic because of the three visual pigments which are sensitive to:**
   a) red, green, and blue
   b) red, yellow, and blue
   c) yellow, green, and blue
   d) red, green, and yellow

2. **The attributes of any color are:**
   a) shade, wavelength, and vibration
   b) chromic wavelength vibration
   c) hue, saturation, and brightness
   d) chromicity, intensity, and vividness

3. **As one stares at a color, it begins to fade. Then, if one quickly looks at a white background, a complementary color will appear. These phenomena are products of:**
   a) fatigue and afterimages
   b) crossed images
   c) wash-out and abnormal retinal correspondence
   d) ectopic phenomenon

4. **If the patient is suspected of having an acquired color vision defect, all of the following apply *except*:**
   a) test each eye separately
   b) the defect tends to remain stable over time
   c) he or she will tend to make color errors scattered all across the color wheel
   d) they can resolve

5. **The condition where all three cone pigments are present but one of the pigment levels is deficient is known as a(n):**
   a) anisochromatism
   b) deutan
   c) protan
   d) anomalous trichromat

6. **If the patient has some difficulty distinguishing blue-green and blue-yellow, the defect would be:**
   a) protanopia
   b) deuteranomaly
   c) tritanomaly
   d) tritanopia

7. **The most common X-linked recessive inheritance pattern resulting in a confusion between red and green (but red is normally bright) is known as:**
   a) deuteranomaly
   b) protanomaly
   c) deuteranopia
   d) protanopia

8. **If a woman is a carrier of the deuteranopia color defect, the odds that she will have a son with the resulting color vision defect is:**
   a) 0.5%
   b) 5%
   c) 35%
   d) 50%

9. **A classic "red-green color defect" is associated with:**
   a) protanomaly
   b) deuteranomaly
   c) anomalous trichromatism
   d) none of the above

10. **Protanopia, deuteranopia, and tritanopia are all examples of:**
    a) trichromatism
    b) dichromatism
    c) monochromatism
    d) anomalous trichromatism

11. **The frequency of dichromatism in the population is:**
    a) 0.5%
    b) 1%
    c) 2%
    d) 5%

12. **A protanope might wear red socks, thinking they are actually:**
    a) yellow
    b) green
    c) blue
    d) black

13. **In blue cone monochromatism, the patient:**
    a) is missing the blue visual pigment
    b) has only the blue visual pigment
    c) has only rod cells
    d) sees only green

14. **Which of the following apply to rod monochromatism?**
    a) patients usually have normal acuity but no color vision
    b) patients generally have nystagmus and photophobia
    c) the fundus appears abnormal
    d) none of the above

15. **Which of the following apply to cone monochromatism?**
    a) patients have no cone photoreceptors
    b) patients generally have good hue discrimination
    c) patients generally have normal acuity
    d) all of the above

16. **The term achromatopsia refers to:**
    a) the absence of any color pigment
    b) a red-green color defect
    c) those who fail the Ishihara plates
    d) total colorblindness

17. **The most common type of anomaloscope is used to quantify:**
    a) red-green abnormalities
    b) blue-yellow abnormalities
    c) protanomaly vs protanopia
    d) deuteranomaly vs deuteranopia

18. **When testing with the anomaloscope, the patient is asked to:**
    a) turn a knob until both halves of the colored circle match in hue
    b) set the color of a circle which the examiner must match
    c) tell the examiner when the colors just begin to be mismatched
    d) tell which half of the circle has the brighter hue

19. **On the anomaloscope, the matching range for a patient with normal color vision:**
    a) does not follow a certain pattern
    b) is very narrow
    c) is very broad
    d) is difficult to interpret

20. **On testing with the anomaloscope, the patient erroneously adds more red to the lower circle to match a yellow test target. The defect demonstrated is:**
    a) deutan
    b) tritan
    c) protanomaly
    d) protan

21. **Which of the following is true regarding testing with the Nagal anomaloscope?**
    a) the patient is tested binocularly
    b) the patient may need spectacle correction
    c) the patient may be dilated
    d) all of the above

22. **When using the Nagal anomaloscope, between each testing situation:**
    a) the patient is dark adapted
    b) the patient closes his or her eyes
    c) the patient looks into the distance to relax accommodation
    d) the patient's retina is slightly "bleached" by having him or her look at a white light

23. **The Farnsworth-Munsell 100-hue test would be useful if one wished to know:**
    a) whether a defect was protan, deutan, or tritan
    b) whether a defect was a protanomaly or protanopia
    c) the severity of a defect
    d) whether a defect was a deuteranomaly or deuteranopia

24. **Which of the following are true regarding the Farnsworth-Munsell 100-hue test?**
    a) it is time-consuming
    b) each of the defect types show arrangement errors along specific axes
    c) the patient with overall poor color discrimination has no definite pattern
    d) all of the above

25. **The Desaturated 15-panel color vision test may detect:**
    a) subtle defects missed by the Farnsworth-Munsell D-15 panel
    b) protanomaly vs protanopia
    c) only gross defects
    d) defects in small children

26. **One of the few tests available for achromatopsia is the:**
    a) Sloan achromatopsia test
    b) pseudoachromatic plates
    c) yarn-matching test
    d) Nagal anomaloscope

Chapter 5

Advanced Clinical Optics

1. **The stenopaic slit might be advantageous to use on a patient with:**
   a) mixed astigmatism
   b) keratoconus
   c) with-the-rule astigmatism
   d) against-the-rule astigmatism

2. **The first step in using the stenopaic slit is to:**
   a) position the slit
   b) enter the axis and power of the patient's cylinder
   c) select a base spherical lens
   d) fog the patient

3. **The patient has moved the stenopaic slit into a position where she states that the letters on the chart look the clearest. This corresponds to:**
   a) the minus cylinder axis
   b) the plus cylinder axis
   c) the axis of lenticular astigmatism
   d) the axis of the steepest K

4. **The stenopaic slit was positioned at 135 degrees with a power of –3.75 for clearest vision. In your second step, you position the slit at 45 degrees and find a power of –9.25. The resulting refractometric measurement is:**
   a)   3.75   5.50   135
   b)   3.75   9.25   135
   c)   3.75   9.25   135
   d)   9.25   5.50   045

5. **Factors which automated refractometers have had to overcome include:**
   a) poor patient acceptance
   b) mixed astigmatism
   c) lenticular astigmatism
   d) none of the above

6. **Most automated refractometers generally operate on the principles of:**
   a) the optometer
   b) photokeratoscopy
   c) retinoscopy
   d) keratometry

7. **Automated refractometers that use infrared lights to measure the refractive error must incorporate:**
   a) a formula to convert the measurement from focusing infrared to focusing visible light
   b) a filter to protect the patient from the harmful effects of infrared light
   c) an infrared target
   d) a laser interferometer

8. **A phoropter equipped with a remote control or a patient response button would be an example of:**
   a) subjective automated refractometry
   b) objective automated refractometry
   c) super-automated refractometry
   d) self-verifying automated refractometry

9. **The best method of measuring the refractive error of most patients is:**
   a) automated
   b) objective
   c) subjective
   d) combined objective and subjective

10. **Subjective refractometry would be most useful in patients with:**
    a) poor verbal skills
    b) anterior segment disease
    c) poor interpretive skills
    d) none of the above

11. **Label each of the four following statements as an advantage of:**
    a) subjective refractometric methods, or
    b) objective refractometric methods

    less likely to prescribe "uncomfortable" glasses
    revelation of latent hyperopia
    reveals information about the media
    eliminates problems created by patient misunderstanding

12. **When performing refractometry on a low vision patient and the distant chart has been moved to 5 feet from the patient:**
    a) retinoscopy is not valid
    b) a change of −0.66 should be made to the final measurement to account for accommodation at this distance
    c) a change of +0.66 should be made to the final measurement to account for accommodation at this distance
    d) the measurement may be used directly

13. **You are performing refractometry on a patient whose low vision is due to nystagmus. You should:**
    a) use a +6.00 lens to fog the other eye
    b) tilt the phoropter toward the patient's left shoulder
    c) turn the phoropter toward the patient's right
    d) occlude one eye as usual

14. **The best instrument to use when measuring the refractive error of a low vision patient is:**
    a) trial lenses and trial frame
    b) phoropter
    c) automated refractometer
    d) prisms to create separate images for each eye

15. **When assessing the near add for a low vision patient, use task-oriented reading material and make sure to:**
    a) keep the reading material at the established distance of 14 inches
    b) move the reading material into the focal distance for each lens
    c) use only isolated optotype reading cards
    d) use a reading stand at 10 inches for every lens

16. **If low vision is due, at least in part, to an irregular corneal surface, the following might be utilized for a better refractometric measurement:**
    a) encourage the patient to blink frequently
    b) artificial tears
    c) a plano soft contact lens
    d) a Soper lens

17. **Given an object located 50 cm from a –3.00 D lens. Where is the image?**
    a) 0.20 cm and on the opposite side from the object
    b) 5.03 cm and on the same side as the object
    c) 20.0 cm and on the same side as the object
    d) 0.20 cm and on the same side as the object

18. **Given an object located 2 m from a +6.50 lens. Where is the image?**
    a) 0.16 cm on the same side as the object
    b) 16 cm on the opposite side from the object
    c) 16 m on the opposite side from the object
    d) 14 cm on the opposite side from the object

19. **Given an object located 3 m from a lens. The image is 25 cm on the opposite side from the object. What is the power of the lens?**
    a) +0.23 D
    b) +4.35 D
    c) +3.70 D
    d) 0.23 D

20. **Given a –2.75 lens. The image is located 12.0 cm from the lens (between the lens and the object). How far away is the object?**
    a) 12.5 m
    b) 12.5 cm
    c) 18 cm
    d) 11.1 m

21. **Given a +4.00 D lens and a +1 D lens, with 25 cm between them. Light from an object 50 cm away from the +4.00 lens enters that lens first. The image will be:**
    a) 0.75 m behind the second lens
    b) 30.3 cm behind the second lens
    c) 5 cm in front of the second lens
    d) 20 cm behind the second lens

22. **Given a +2.00 D lens and a –8.00 D lens, with 37 cm between them. Light from an object 4.0 m away first enters the +2.00 lens. The image will be:**
    a) 70 cm behind the +2.00 lens
    b) 33 cm in front of the   8.00 lens
    c) 57 cm behind the +2.00 lens
    d) 20 cm behind the   8.00 lens

23. **The power of a plane (flat) mirror is:**
    a) dependent on the amount of divergence
    b) dependent on the amount of convergence
    c) dependent on its distance from the reflected object
    d) plano (zero)

24. **A plane (flat) mirror creates an image that is:**
    a) virtual, erect, but not inverted from side to side
    b) real, erect, but not inverted from side to side
    c) virtual, inverted, and single
    d) real, inverted, and the image is on the opposite side

25. **You are looking straight at yourself in a plane (flat) mirror from 1 m away. The image of yourself appears to be:**
    a) 1 m away
    b) 1.5 m away
    c) 2.0 m away
    d) 0.5 m away

26. **The law of reflection (the angle of incidence equals the angle of reflection) applies to:**
    a) plane (flat) mirrors
    b) convex mirrors
    c) concave mirrors
    d) all mirrors

27. **A curved mirror with a minified, virtual image on the opposite side from the object also has:**
    a) no vergence
    b) negative vergence
    c) positive vergence
    d) mixed vergence

28. **Given that real images are inverted, the image seen in a shaving mirror is erect if:**
    a) the mirror is mounted upside down
    b) the mirror is convex
    c) you are farther back than the mirror's focal distance
    d) you are closer than the mirror's focal distance

29. **The radius of curvature of a concave mirror is 100 mm. What is the power of the mirror?**
    a) +20 D
    b)   20 D
    c) +50 D
    d) +0.05 D

30. **What is the focal length of a –50 D convex mirror?**
    a) 0.04 m
    b) 0.2 m
    c) 25 m
    d) 1.2 m

31. **The warning "Caution: Images are closer than they appear" would appear on which type of mirror?**
    a) plane (flat)
    b) concave
    c) convex
    d) none of the above

32. **Which of the following is measured in diopters?**
    a) range of accommodation
    b) near point
    c) angle kappa
    d) accommodative amplitude

33. **Range of accommodation is defined as the eye's:**
    a) focal length
    b) depth of focus
    c) relationship of accommodation to convergence
    d) near point

34. **Your patient's near point of accommodation is 8 cm and the far point is 33 cm. This patient's range of accommodation is:**
    a) 4.12 cm
    b) 25 cm
    c) 33 cm
    d) 41 cm

35. **In the patient in Question 34, what is his or her approximate amplitude of accommodation?**
    a) 3.03 D
    b) 12.5 D
    c) 15.5 D
    d) 9.5 D

36. **When using the Prince rule to measure the patient's amplitude of accommodation (with no near add in place), it is a given that:**
    a) any distant refractive error is corrected to emmetropia
    b) any distant refractive error is uncorrected
    c) the near target simulates parallel light rays
    d) a working lens power of +1.50 will be deducted after testing

37. **Your patient is a 55-year-old who is behind the phoropter and corrected for distance with −2.50 sph OU. Her near point when thus corrected to emmetropia is off the 1 m long Prince rule. How can you measure her accommodative amplitude?**
    a) put a +3.00 add into the phoropter and measure; subtract 3 D from the measurement
    b) put a +3.00 add into the phoropter and measure; add 3 D to the measurement
    c) remove the   2.50 and measure; subtract 2.50 from the measurement
    d) pull the card off the rule and hold it farther back from the patient, then walk the card forward until blurring occurs

38. **Normally, the patient's amplitude of accommodation will be about the same in both eyes. Which of the following can cause the amplitudes to be *unequal*?**
    a) monocular pseudophakia
    b) a mistake in the refractometric measurement
    c) trauma
    d) all of the above

39. **Presbyopia generally becomes noticeable around age 40 because:**
    a) the near point has moved up to 25 cm
    b) the near point has receded to 25 cm
    c) the near point has moved up to 15 cm
    d) the near point has receded to 15 cm

40. **Before measuring the patient for the near add, one should perform:**
    a) a cycloplegic refraction
    b) a paraboline test
    c) binocular balancing
    d) near point of convergence

41. **Your patient is 60 years old and has not had an eye exam in 10 years. She has been using a pair of +1.25 readers for desk work, but complains of problems seeing closer than desk level. She refuses a bifocal or trifocal. To read at 14 inches, she requires a +2.25 add. To increase her satisfaction with the new +2.25 reading glasses, you should tell her all of the following *except*:**
    a) she will need to hold reading material closer than what she's been used to
    b) her range of focus will be increased
    c) keep the old glasses for desk work
    d) distant objects will appear even more blurry through the +2.25s

42. **Assuming that the presbyopic patient can still accommodate to some degree, about how much of the patient's own accommodation should be expended for reading, and how much should be provided with an add?**
    a) 50% by the patient and the rest with the add
    b) 25% by the patient and the rest with the add
    c) 75% by the patient and the rest with the add
    d) 100% with the add

43. **A 6X magnifier has what effective dioptric power?**
    a) +6.00 D
    b) +15.00 D
    c) +24.00 D
    d) unable to answer from data given

44. **You are helping a low vision patient with single vision reading glasses. You select a pair with the label 10/12. This means that these glasses:**
    a) have a +10 lens in the right and +12 in the left
    b) are progressives that go from +10 on the top to +12 on the bottom
    c) are +10 D lenses with 12 base in prism diopters
    d) are +10 D lenses with 12 base out prism diopters

45. **Which of the following is *not* true regarding hand magnifiers?**
    a) changing the distance from the eye to the magnifier changes the image size and focus
    b) patients should look through their distance correction when using the magnifier
    c) no accommodation is necessary when using the magnifier
    d) an aspheric design will eliminate distortion at the lens periphery

46. **A monocular telescope is labeled 8   20, 7.5. This translates as:**
    a) 8 times enlargement, 20 mm objective lens diameter, and 7.5 degree field of view
    b) 8 times enlargement, 20 diopters of power, and 7.5 base in prism
    c) 8 degree field of view, 20 diopters of power, and 7.5 mm objective lens diameter
    d) 8 diopters of power, 20 degree field of view, and 7.5 base out prism

47. **The optical system of a telescope produces divergent rays that create a larger retinal image. This scenario is known as:**
    a) relative size magnification
    b) angular magnification
    c) relative distance magnification
    d) projection magnification

48. **Which of the following is *not* true?**
    a) bioptics are attached above the optical axis, and may be used for driving in some states
    b) telemicroscopes are attached below the optical axis, and are used for reading
    c) a makeshift telescope can be created by combining a high plus contact lens with a high minus glasses lens
    d) a patient with a narrow visual field can broaden the field by looking through a telescope backward

49. The formula *induced prism = lens power (D)   optical center displacement (cm)* is referred to as:
   a) Prince's rule
   b) Prentice's rule
   c) Snell's law of induced prism
   d) Lens' law of induced prism

50. The patient's prescription is +6.00 in each eye, and the optical center of the left lens needs to be decentered in order to induce 2 prism diopters base out. How much should the optical center be decentered, and in what direction?
   a) decentered out by 1.2 mm
   b) decentered in by 1.2 mm
   c) decentered out by 3.3 mm
   d) decentered in by 3.3 mm

51. The patient is wearing +2.75 sphere OD and +2.00 sphere OS. The lenses are decentered in by 2.75 mm OD and 1.25 OS. What is the approximate total prismatic effect?
   a) 1.00 prism diopters base in
   b) 0.50 prism diopters base out
   c) 10.0 prism diopters base in
   d) 0.1 prism diopters base out

52. What is the total induced base up prism when the patient looks 3 mm above the optical centers of the following: OD: –3.00 – 2.00   180; OS: –4.50 – 2.25   090.
   a) 2.85 prism diopters
   b) 0.15 prism diopters
   c) 0.975 prism diopters
   d) 0.375 prism diopters

53. A safety lens must be able to withstand the impact of a 1-inch steel ball dropped from 50 inches in order to qualify for:
   a) industrial wear
   b) street wear
   c) sportswear
   d) pediatric wear

54. In order to qualify as an industrial safety lens, a plus lens must be at least this thick in the periphery, and a minus lens must be at least this thick in the middle:
   a) 1 mm
   b) 2.2 mm
   c) 3 mm
   d) 4 mm

55. Which would be the superior safety lens?
   a) plastic hard-resin
   b) polycarbonate
   c) chemically treated impact-resistant glass
   d) a plastic/glass laminate

56. The most widely used concept of the schematic eye was developed by:
a) Copeland
b) Snell
c) Gullstrand
d) Kirby

57. The schematic eye was developed in order to provide:
a) methods of correcting refractive errors
b) the optical constants of the eye
c) information for the development of new instrumentation
d) information for understanding strabismus

58. Examples of the constants established by the schematic eye are:
a) refractive error, astigmatic correction, accommodation
b) numbers of photoreceptor cells, numbers of corneal endothelial cells
c) amount of iris pigment, range of pupillary movements, range of extraocular muscle movement
d) index of refraction, dioptric power, radius of curvature

59. Sturm's interval occurs in:
a) the schematic eye
b) spherocylindrical lens combinations
c) irregular astigmatism
d) cases where prism is induced

60. The focused, conical shape of the light rays within Sturm's interval is known as:
a) the principal cardinal point
b) the nodal point
c) circle of least confusion
d) Sturm's conoid

61. Within Sturm's conoid is an area where vision is clearest. This is known as the:
a) circle of least confusion
b) real image
c) virtual image
d) posterior principal plane

Chapter 6

Advanced Ocular Motility

1. **If amblyopia in a child does not respond to treatment, the amblyopia is referred to as:**
   a) suppressive
   b) organic
   c) functional
   d) dense

2. **A child with uncorrected/undetected high myopia in both eyes may develop:**
   a) reverse amblyopia
   b) reflex amblyopia
   c) refractive amblyopia
   d) anisometropic amblyopia

3. **A child with one myopic eye and one hyperopic eye:**
   a) is guaranteed to develop anisometropic amblyopia
   b) does not have normal fusion while uncorrected
   c) generally develops non-alternating strabismus
   d) does not require refractive correction

4. **In a child with congenital ptosis that obscures the pupil, even after the lid is repaired, it is likely that the child will need to be treated for:**
   a) alternating amblyopia
   b) nocturnal amblyopia
   c) crossed amblyopia
   d) amblyopia ex anopsia

5. **Which of the following is both a cause of amblyopia as well as a sign that amblyopia exists in a particular child patient?**
   a) freely-alternating strabismus
   b) non-alternating strabismus
   c) intermittent strabismus
   d) phoria

6. **A child being patched to treat amblyopia has been faithfully wearing the patch full-time, but has missed the last two appointments. This creates concern that:**
   a) treatment will take longer than necessary
   b) reverse amblyopia will occur
   c) glasses may become necessary
   d) pharmacologic penalization may become necessary

7. **In the mildly myopic child, cycloplegic penalization of the dominant eye as treatment for amblyopia:**
   a) is the best method of treatment
   b) is effective only if cyclopentolate is used
   c) is effective only if atropine ointment is used
   d) is not very useful

8. **When using a conventional stick-on patch to treat amblyopia, all of the following are true** *except*:
   a) it may be applied to either the glasses or directly to the face with equal results
   b) wearing the patch during sleep does not count as treatment time
   c) the younger the child, the more frequent the follow-up
   d) there are psychological factors to consider

9. **A Bangerter foil of 0.4 would be used when:**
   a) vision in the amblyopic eye is 20/50 or worse
   b) the child is young and has previously accepted conventional patching
   c) the vision in the two eyes is only a few lines different and persistent
   d) the vision in the two eyes is vastly different and persistent

10. **On which amblyopic patient would the full amount of plus correction generally be prescribed?**
    a) every amblyopic patient with a refractive error
    b) the patient with an esodeviation
    c) the patient with an exodeviation
    d) the patient who is ortho

11. **A 4-year-old patient has been successfully treated for amblyopia and now has equal vision in both eyes. The parents may be told that:**
    a) their problems and worries are over
    b) it is not guaranteed that optimal vision will be maintained
    c) there will be a definite need for future treatment
    d) the child may require further treatment around puberty

12. **In the child with strabismic amblyopia, optimizing the vision in the amblyopic eye is generally attempted:**
    a) prior to any alignment surgery
    b) following any alignment surgery
    c) instead of alignment surgery
    d) by using glasses only

13. **If the child has a high, uncorrected astigmatism, the following might develop:**
    a) color amblyopia
    b) suppression amblyopia
    c) meridional amblyopia
    d) isoametropia

14. **Which of the following muscles does *not* originate at the annulus of Zinn?**
    a) inferior oblique
    b) superior oblique
    c) lateral rectus
    d) inferior rectus

15. **The configuration created by the insertion of the rectus muscles into the globe is known as:**
    a) Meyer's loop
    b) Circle of Willis
    c) the spiral of Tillaux
    d) Ridley's circle

16. **Each EOM runs directly from its origin to connect to the globe *except* the:**
    a) inferior oblique
    b) superior oblique
    c) superior rectus
    d) inferior rectus

17. **When the eye is in primary position, the muscle planes of which muscles coincide with the visual axis?**
    a) superior and inferior recti
    b) superior and inferior obliques
    c) lateral and medial recti
    d) superior oblique and inferior rectus

18. **Which of the following EOMs insert behind the equator?**
    a) SO and IO
    b) SR and LR
    c) LR and MR
    d) SR and IR

19. **The lateral rectus is innervated by which nerve?**
    a) inferior division of the oculomotor nerve
    b) trochlear
    c) superior division of the oculomotor nerve
    d) abducens

20. **Which muscle is innervated by the superior division of CNIII?**
    a) superior rectus
    b) medial rectus
    c) inferior rectus
    d) inferior oblique

21. **The law that states that an equal amount of innervation goes to the yoke muscles of each eye is:**
    a) Herring's law
    b) Sherrington's law
    c) Panum's law
    d) Snell's law

22. You are evaluating ductions of the right eye and direct the patient to look to the left. To do this, the MR must contract and the LR must relax. The law that applies to this occurrence is:
    a) Herring's law
    b) Sherrington's law
    c) Panum's law
    d) Snell's law

23. You are conducting a binocular range of motion test and direct the patient to look up and right. Which law says that the RSR and LIO are receiving the same amount of stimulation?
    a) Herring's law
    b) Sherrington's law
    c) Panum's law
    d) Snell's law

24. You note that the patient has a right esotropia due to a lateral rectus palsy, greater when OD is fixing. The fact that the secondary deviation is greater than the primary deviation is a product of:
    a) Herring's law
    b) Sherrington's law
    c) Panum's law
    d) Snell's law

25. For each diopter of accommodation expended by the patient, there is a correlated change in:
    a) pupil size
    b) angle kappa
    c) corneal reflex
    d) convergence

26. A comparison of the amount of convergence (in prism diopters) to the amount of accommodation (in diopters) is known as:
    a) accommodative convergence/accommodation ratio
    b) accommodative prism/diopter ratio
    c) near point of convergence
    d) near point of accommodation

27. Which of the following is *not* true regarding the AC/A ratio?
    a) it varies among individuals, but generally remains fixed for life (barring intervention)
    b) age affects accommodation but not accommodative convergence
    c) an AC/A of 3/1 to 6/1 is considered normal
    d) a child with a high AC/A ratio will probably be treated with a bifocal

28. Given: A normal, emmetropic patient must accommodate 3 D to see an object at 1/3 m, and that 18 prism diopters of convergence is also required at this distance. If a patient with an AC/A of 8/1 is looking at an object 1/3 of a meter away, how many extra diopters of convergence will he exhibit?
    a) 42 prism diopters
    b) 24 prism diopters
    c) 6 prism diopters
    d) 3 prism diopters

29. Which patient must exert effort to control convergence at distance, even in the presence of a normal AC/A?
    a) uncorrected myope
    b) emmetrope
    c) corrected hyperope
    d) uncorrected hyperope

30. Your patient (who is corrected to emmetropia) has an esodeviation of 35 prism diopters when looking at an accommodative target 1/3 m away. When you introduce a +3.00 lens to this system, the esodeviation diminishes to 14 prism diopters. What is the patient's AC/A?
    a) 7/1
    b) 16/1
    c) 3/1
    d) 21/1

31. You have already tested your patient for EOM deviations, and there was no movement on cover testing. Now your patient is fixating on a penlight that you are shining straight at his right eye from 1/3 m away. If the reflex falls directly on the pupillary center, this indicates:
    a) a normal angle kappa
    b) a positive angle kappa
    c) an angle kappa of 2 to 4 degrees
    d) an angle kappa of zero

32. You have already tested your patient for EOM deviations, and there was no movement on cover testing. Your patient is now fixating on a penlight that you are shining straight at his right eye, and you find a negative angle kappa. This will give the false impression of:
    a) esotropia
    b) exotropia
    c) hypertropia
    d) hypotropia

33. A positive angle kappa may mask a(n):
    a) exotropia
    b) esotropia
    c) hypertropia
    d) hypotropia

34. **The actual measurement of the angle kappa may be done by using:**
    a) prism diopters rule
    b) Prince's rule
    c) a perimeter or synoptophore slide
    d) keratometer

35. **A patient's ability to overcome induced prism in his or her glasses is a product of his or her:**
    a) AC/A
    b) angle kappa
    c) fusional amplitudes
    d) suppression

36. **Which of the following fusional amplitudes are strongest in the normal patient?**
    a) convergence at distance
    b) convergence at near
    c) divergence at distance
    d) divergence at near

37. **When testing fusional amplitudes, the prism that first causes diplopia is recorded as the:**
    a) break point
    b) recovery point
    c) doubling point
    d) maximum prism

38. **Which of the following is *not* true regarding stereopsis?**
    a) its influence is diminished beyond 20 feet
    b) it is based on horizontal disparity
    c) if binocular vision and fusion are present, stereopsis exists as well
    d) it does not have a motor component

39. **To avoid exam contamination, the following tests should be performed in which order?**
    a) Worth 4 dot, cover-uncover, visual acuity, stereoacuity
    b) stereoacuity, Worth 4 dot, cover-uncover, visual acuity
    c) visual acuity, cover-uncover, Worth 4 dot, stereoacuity
    d) cover-uncover, stereoacuity, visual acuity, Worth 4 dot

40. **Central stereopsis (or fine stereopsis) takes place:**
    a) in the presence of abnormal retinal correspondence
    b) even in monocular patients
    c) at the foveae
    d) at the foveae and in the peripheral retina

41. **Given that the Titmus test is set for a test distance of 15 inches, what will be the disparity of the 40 second set of test circles if the test booklet is held at 30 inches?**
    a) 40 seconds
    b) 80 seconds
    c) 20 seconds
    d) 10 seconds

42. **Nystagmus movements where the movements are equal in speed, equal in amplitude, and have equal duration in each direction are referred to as:**
    a) jerk
    b) spasmus nutans
    c) pendular
    d) congenital

43. **Which of the following *cannot* be elicited in the normal patient?**
    a) end point nystagmus
    b) latent nystagmus
    c) optokinetic nystagmus
    d) stimulation of semicircular canals

44. **Adult-onset nystagmus will frequently cause the patient to complain of:**
    a) diplopia
    b) oscillopsia
    c) photophobia
    d) extraocular muscle pain

45. **Which of the following is *not* true regarding congenital nystagmus?**
    a) it is often associated with maternal infections
    b) the child may adopt a specific head position
    c) the child will frequently outgrow the condition
    d) it is often associated with visual impairment and/or lesions in the optic system

46. **The root cause of nystagmus is thought to be:**
    a) fixation confusion due to eccentric fixation
    b) extraocular muscle imbalances due to neurological defect(s)
    c) "searching" movements by eyes with poor vision
    d) a neurological feedback problem that results in poor control of the fixation mechanism

47. **Which of the following is the result of continuous muscle contractions of the eye at rest?**
    a) tonic convergence
    b) proximal convergence
    c) accommodative convergence
    d) fusional convergence

48. **Which of the following best describes divergence?**
    a) it is a voluntary action
    b) it is linked to accommodation
    c) it occurs as the globes return to a parallel position following convergence
    d) it is stronger at near

49. **An orthophoric patient complains that when he's looking at an object at near, objects beyond that are doubled. He's describing:**
    a) faulty stereopsis
    b) crossed diplopia
    c) physiologic diplopia
    d) uncrossed diplopia

50. **Which of the following is true regarding the horopter?**
    a) it represents the locus of all object points that fall on corresponding retinal points
    b) points on the horopter appear as single (ie, not doubled)
    c) it is horizontal, not vertical
    d) all of the above

51. **The small area in front of and behind the horopter where single vision is present is known as the:**
    a) circle of least confusion
    b) conoid of Sturm
    c) Panum's area
    d) Hubbard's area

52. **The horizontal area of Panum's fusional space:**
    a) stays the same in all areas
    b) increases as you approach the periphery
    c) decreases as you approach the periphery
    d) expands vertically

53. **Why is an orthophoric person normally unaware of physiologic diplopia?**
    a) physiologic amblyopia
    b) we have learned to disregard it
    c) it is too blurred to be distinguished as double
    d) it involves non-macular photoreceptors

54. **Retinal correspondence is one feature necessary in order to achieve:**
    a) foveal fixation
    b) normal ocular motility
    c) similar retinal images
    d) binocular vision

55. **An orthophoric patient with normal binocular vision will perceive an object as being in the same point in space when viewed with either eye because of:**
    a) overlapping fields
    b) retinal correspondence
    c) monocular clues
    d) depth perception

56. **If retinal points which are normally non-corresponding develop a correspondence, this situation is known as:**
    a) harmonious retinal correspondence
    b) abnormal retinal correspondence
    c) suppression of correspondence
    d) strabismic correspondence

57. **Which of the following is *not* true regarding abnormal retinal correspondence?**
    a) the patient is still able to exhibit fine stereopsis
    b) it is, at best, a rudimentary form of binocular vision
    c) once established, it does not respond well to treatment
    d) it is an adaptive process

58. **Which of the following would indicate exotropia associated with convergence insufficiency?**
    a) distance deviation = 15 prism diopters, near deviation = 30 prism diopters
    b) distance deviation = 15 prism diopters, near deviation = 15 prism diopters
    c) distance deviation = 15 prism diopters, near deviation = 0 prism diopters (orthophoric)
    d) distance deviation = 30 prism diopters, near deviation = 15 prism diopters

59. **Patient complaints associated with convergence insufficiency include:**
    a) headaches after prolonged periods of looking into the distance
    b) letters on street signs jumping/swimming
    c) closing one eye to watch a movie at the theater
    d) falling asleep after several minutes of reading

60. **Patients with combined convergence insufficiency and accommodative insufficiency:**
    a) do not respond well to conventional orthoptic exercises
    b) respond well to surgical correction and reading glasses
    c) respond well to pharmacologic treatment
    d) respond well to base out prism and reading glasses

61. **Which of the following would indicate exotropia associated with divergence excess?**
    a) distance deviation = 30 prism diopters, near deviation = 45 prism diopters
    b) distance deviation = 0 prism diopters (orthophoric), near deviation = 15 prism diopters
    c) distance deviation = 45 prism diopters, near deviation = 30 prism diopters
    d) distance deviation = 30 prism diopters, near deviation = 30 prism diopters

62. **You believe you have discovered an exotropia due to divergence excess. To make sure that you are not dealing with pseudo-divergence excess, you should:**
    a) repeat the near measurement through +3.00 D lenses
    b) repeat the distance measurement through +3.00 lenses
    c) repeat the near measurement through   3.00 lenses
    d) repeat the distance measurement through   3.00 lenses

63. **An adult has suddenly developed an esotropia at distance (orthophoria at near) with no history of head trauma and no neurological disease. This scenario describes:**
    a) Duane syndrome
    b) divergence paralysis
    c) divergence insufficiency
    d) convergence insufficiency

64. **Initial therapy of convergence insufficiency consists of:**
    a) bilateral LR resections
    b) a reading add
    c) base in prisms
    d) base out prisms

65. **Alternate cover testing on a patient with dissociated vertical deviation (DVD) reveals that:**
    a) one or both eyes drifts down under the cover
    b) one or both eyes drifts up under the cover
    c) one eye drifts up under the cover and the other eye drifts down under the cover
    d) an eye will alternately drift down, then up under the cover

66. **Which of the following is *not* true regarding DVD?**
    a) the deviation may decrease if occlusion of the eye is prolonged
    b) the deviation is not always equal between the two eyes
    c) when the cover is removed the eye may overshoot before settling at the midline
    d) it may be manifest when the patient is tired

67. **Your patient has a DVD in both eyes, and you are doing a red glass test. The red image will appear:**
    a) above the fixation light when either eye looks through the red glass
    b) below the fixation light when either eye looks through the red glass
    c) one above and one below, depending on which eye is looking through the red glass
    d) as a single pink light

68. **Which of the following is true regarding DVD?**
    a) it is seen in children more often than adults
    b) there is disagreement as to its etiology
    c) it is sometimes confused with overaction of the inferior obliques
    d) all of the above

69. **Strabismus in Graves' disease is generally caused by:**
    a) restriction of movement
    b) decreasing nerve stimuli
    c) loss of muscle tone
    d) muscle paralysis

70. **Your patient is a cooperative young child who obviously has a horizontal deviation. During range of motion testing, you notice that when attempting ADduction, the fissure of her left eye narrows and the eye itself retracts. This suggests that the child has:**
    a) Brown syndrome
    b) Goldenhar syndrome
    c) Duane syndrome
    d) superior oblique myokymia

71. **You are checking range of motion on a cooperative young child and notice that in ADduction the left eye does not seem to elevate well. You also notice that when the child is simply sitting in the chair talking to you, he has a chin-up head position. This scenario suggests that the child has:**
    a) weakness of the inferior oblique
    b) Brown syndrome
    c) superior oblique myokymia
    d) Crouzon syndrome

72. **Your patient is an aphasic but fairly cooperative elderly man who has been brought to the office by a nursing home attendant. The nursing home records state that the patient is diabetic. You note a ptosis on the right, and that the right eye is rotated down and out. What test can you perform to help determine whether or not you are dealing with a diabetic third nerve palsy?**
    a) pupillary exam
    b) forced ductions
    c) prism and cover
    d) Worth 4 dot

73. **Which of the following is *not* true regarding monofixation syndrome?**
    a) there is central suppression of the non-preferred eye during binocular gaze
    b) the patient is usually emmetropic
    c) the deviation is small during the cover-uncover test, but tends to increase on prism and alternate cover test
    d) stereopsis is 67 seconds or less

Chapter 7

Advanced Photography

1. **If, after absorbing energy, the molecules of a material are excited and light is emitted when they return to a ground state, this is termed:**
   a) electromagnetic spectrum
   b) luminescence
   c) gamma radiation
   d) incandescence

2. **If luminescence stops after the exciting light has been removed, this is termed:**
   a) hypofluorescence
   b) incandescence
   c) phosphorescence
   d) fluorescence

3. **Blood that has been mixed with fluorescein will glow when excited by the appropriate wavelength of light because then the fluorescein:**
   a) absorbs blue light and emits yellow-green light
   b) absorbs green light and emits yellow light
   c) absorbs all light except blue
   d) reflects all light except yellow-green

4. **Fluorescein angiography is which type of test?**
   a) diagnostic
   b) subjective
   c) radiation
   d) ultrasonic

5. **The blue filter that excites the fluorescein to emit a higher wavelength is:**
   a) barrier filter
   b) Wratten filter
   c) diffuser
   d) exciter filter

6. **The barrier filter:**
   a) absorbs unwanted blue (exciter) light
   b) is red
   c) is used to take the monochromatic (red-free) photo
   d) is not needed during the "late phase" of an angiogram

7. **When looking at a control photo, aging filters can be detected by the:**
   a) lack of detail
   b) autofluorescence of the optic nerve
   c) visibility of blood vessels
   d) blank frame

8. **If the exciter filter is worn out, one must:**
   a) stop the fluorescein study immediately
   b) use a slower film to capture the image
   c) simply replace the exciter filter
   d) replace both the exciter and the barrier filters

9. **Prior to taking the control photos, one must:**
    a) dilate the pupils
    b) loosen the tourniquet
    c) start the camera's timer
    d) all of the above

10. **A photograph is taken prior to dye injection using a green filter in order to:**
    a) document any pseudofluorescence
    b) provide a clinical representation of the subject
    c) make sure the camera has film in it
    d) identify the patient's face

11. **The first step in a fluorescein dye study is:**
    a) patient education and informed consent
    b) applying a tourniquet
    c) disinfecting the patient's skin
    d) selecting the injection site

12. **The side effects or complications of fluorescein dye injection include:**
    a) yellowish skin and urine
    b) nausea and vomiting
    c) infiltration
    d) all of the above

13. **The actual act of injecting the fluorescein should start when the:**
    a) IV needle is inserted
    b) photographer is ready
    c) tourniquet has been tightened
    d) patient gives the go-ahead

14. **The film generally used to record fluorescein angiograms is:**
    a) b&w print ISO 400
    b) b&w print ISO 100
    c) color print film, ISO 400
    d) color slide film, ISO 400

15. **The average arm-to-retina circulation time from a rapid dye push is:**
    a) 2 to 8 seconds
    b) 10 to 20 seconds
    c) 30 to 40 seconds
    d) 45 to 60 seconds

16. **Number the fluorescein phases in order of their occurrence:**
    capillary phase
    full venous flow
    choroidal flush
    late phase
    arterial phase
    early venous phase with laminar flow

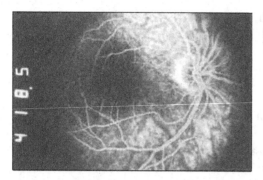

Figure 7-1. (Reprinted with permission from Cunningham D. *Clinical Ocular Photography.* Thorofare, NJ: SLACK Incorporated; 1998.)

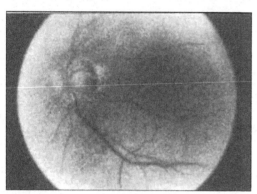

Figure 7-2. (Reprinted with permission from Cunningham D. *Clinical Ocular Photography.* Thorofare, NJ: SLACK Incorporated; 1998.)

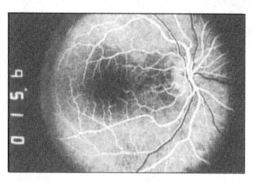

Figure 7-3. (Reprinted with permission from Cunningham D. *Clinical Ocular Photography.* Thorofare, NJ: SLACK Incorporated; 1998.)

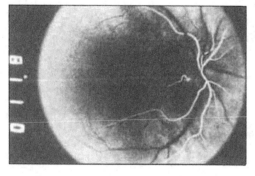

Figure 7-4. (Reprinted with permission from Cunningham D. *Clinical Ocular Photography.* Thorofare, NJ: SLACK Incorporated; 1998.)

17. **Match the photographs (Figures 7-1 through 7-4) to the correct phase:**
    a) choroidal flush
    b) arterial phase
    c) laminar flow
    d) full venous phase

18. **The "late shots" are taken:**
    a) 2 minutes after injection
    b) 5 minutes after injection
    c) 10 minutes after injection
    d) 60 minutes after injection

19. **Leakage from a retinal blood vessel will manifest as:**
    a) hypophosphorescence
    b) hyperphosphorescence
    c) hypofluorescence
    d) hyperfluorescence

20. **If a retinal blood vessel is occluded, this will be manifest as:**
    a) hyperincandescence
    b) hypoincandescence
    c) hyperfluorescence
    d) hypofluorescence

21. **If there is blood present outside of the retinal blood vessels (as in a vitreous hemorrhage), this will be manifest as:**
    a) hypofluorescence
    b) hyperfluorescence
    c) extravasation
    d) autofluorescence

22. **A "window defect" occurs due to:**
    a) a laser scan
    b) an area where pigment is lacking in the retinal pigment epithelium
    c) an area of neovascularization
    d) a leaking retinal blood vessel

23. **When performing slit lamp photography, a photograph of the eye using low magnification and diffuse lighting is recommended to:**
    a) judge the patient's tolerance to the flash
    b) judge the corneal reflection
    c) provide identification
    d) provide orientation

24. **By convention as well as for ease of use, the illuminator in slit lamp photography is usually positioned:**
    a) nasally
    b) temporally
    c) temporally for OD and nasally for OS
    d) nasally for OD and temporally for OS

25. **When taking a slit lamp photo, if one wished to highlight the contours of an iris tumor, the illumination technique of choice would be:**
    a) tangential
    b) diffuse
    c) pinpoint
    d) retroillumination

26. **If one was to take a slit lamp photograph of a cortical spoking cataract, an effective illumination technique would be:**
    a) tangential
    b) diffuse
    c) pinpoint
    d) retroillumination

27. **The standard type of film used in slit lamp photography is:**
    a) color print film
    b) color slide film
    c) b&w slide film
    d) b&w print film

28. **External photographs taken prior to strabismus surgery will include (at a minimum):**
    a) upgaze, downgaze, and primary positions
    b) a head shot, primary position, and worm's eye view
    c) nine positions of gaze plus a head shot
    d) right gaze, left gaze, primary position, plus a head shot

29. **The patient has given verbal agreement to be a model in before and after photographs of a blepharoplasty. In order to display the full head shots, you will need:**
    a) a standardized background
    b) to just eliminate the patient's name from the display
    c) enlargements of the photos
    d) the patient's written consent

30. **An external photograph taken of both eyes is generally at which degree of magnification?**
    a) 1:10
    b) 1:4
    c) 1:7
    d) 1:1

31. **To increase the subject-to-camera distance for external photography, one may use a:**
    a) 105 mm (long focal length) lens
    b) 50 mm (normal) lens
    c) 20 mm (short focal length) lens
    d) 14 mm (fish-eye) lens

32. **To reduce the reflection of the flash in the patient's cornea (and thus on the photograph), the flash unit of choice is a:**
    a) bracket-mounted flash with a large reflector
    b) point source flash
    c) ring light
    d) hand-held point flash with a large reflector

33. **Specular microscopy is used to evaluate the:**
    a) corneal epithelium
    b) corneal endothelium
    c) corneal stroma
    d) anterior chamber angle

34. **Videotape is frequently used in specular microscopy because:**
    a) the microscope uses such high magnification
    b) individual frames can be photographed later
    c) individual frames can be "frozen" for evaluation
    d) all of the above

35. **In addition to the quality of the cells viewed with specular microscopy, the number of cells are calculated by using:**
    a) an overlay grid
    b) a computer program
    c) template cards
    d) all of the above

36. **The developer is used to:**
    a) wash the film
    b) halt the conversion of silver halides
    c) convert the silver halides in the film into metallic silver
    d) convert the metallic silver in the film to silver halides

37. **The stop bath is used to:**
    a) enhance the film image
    b) speed the action of the developer
    c) fix the image on the film
    d) halt the action of the developer

38. **The film may be safely exposed to light:**
    a) when it is removed from the cassette
    b) after using the developer
    c) after using the stop bath
    d) after using the fixer

39. **Once the developer is poured into the tank, the tank should be tapped a few times in order to:**
    a) mix it well
    b) activate the chemicals
    c) eliminate bubbles
    d) ensure that the film is totally immersed

40. **Developer may be diluted with water in a 1:1 ratio in order to easily reach the proper temperature; however, one must then:**
    a) change the developing time according to manufacturer's recommendations
    b) double the developing time
    c) decrease the strength of the stop bath
    d) double the amount of developer used

41. **In addition to the factors of volume and temperature of solutions and time of development, another important factor in the developing stage of film processing is:**
    a) agitation
    b) proper light exposure
    c) excitation of the molecules
    d) barometric pressure in the lab

Chapter 8

Advanced Pharmacology

1. **The ability of a drug to remain in its active form over a period of time refers to its:**
   a) tonicity
   b) stability
   c) expiration
   d) all of the above

2. **The degradation of a drug may be furthered by:**
   a) light
   b) moisture
   c) heat
   d) all of the above

3. **Antioxidants are sometimes added to solutions in order to:**
   a) increase the vitamin value of the medication
   b) help reduce oxidants in the ocular tissues
   c) help reduce the degradation of a drug by oxygen
   d) act as an anti-microbial agent

4. **Solutions tend to be more stable if they are:**
   a) pH neutral
   b) slightly alkaline (basic)
   c) slightly acidic
   d) slightly saline

5. **The pH of a topical ocular medication plays a key role in patient compliance by affecting the drug's:**
   a) viscosity
   b) saline balance
   c) tolerance
   d) shelf-life

6. **If the pH of an ocular solution is 8.5:**
   a) it will sting on installation because it is alkaline
   b) it will sting on installation because it is acidic
   c) it will sting on installation because it is neutral
   d) it will not sting because it is compatible with the pH of the tear film

7. **In order to place the pH of an ocular solution into the tolerated range, the manufacturer may add:**
   a) preservatives
   b) buffers
   c) sterile saline
   d) litmus agents

8. **The concentration of a drug as it affects the osmotic pressure balance on the eye is referred to as:**
   a) tonicity
   b) viscosity
   c) molecular weight
   d) strength

9. **A drug is less irritating to the eye if it is isotonic with:**
   a) other drops the patient is using
   b) aqueous
   c) the tear film
   d) water

10. **A topical hypertonic drug might be used on the eye:**
    a) to hydrate the tissues
    b) to rinse the tissues
    c) to push water into the tissues
    d) to draw water out of the tissues

11. **A systemic hypertonic drug that might be used to treat angle-closure glaucoma is:**
    a) pilocarpine
    b) glycerin
    c) normal saline
    d) Ringers lactate

12. **A topical ophthalmic drug preparation is considered unsterile:**
    a) once it is opened
    b) only if it touches the lashes or lids
    c) only if bacteria can be cultured from it
    d) none of the above

13. **Chemicals that are added to ophthalmic drugs to reduce or eliminate organism contamination are known as:**
    a) buffers
    b) disinfectants
    c) preservatives
    d) virusides

14. **The two classes of preservatives are:**
    a) bacteriostatic and bacteriocidal
    b) organic and non-organic
    c) buffered and non-buffered
    d) disinfectants and sterilants

15. **A common preservative currently in popular use is:**
    a) thimerosal
    b) bensalkonium chloride
    c) tetrahydrozoline
    d) phenylephrine

16. **Tingling in the extremities as a result of taking acetazolamide is an example of a(n):**
    a) drug interaction
    b) anaphylactic shock
    c) allergy
    d) side effect

17. **Common signs and symptoms of a topical allergic reaction to ocular medication include:**
    a) rash, itching, redness, and swelling
    b) pain, redness, and discharge
    c) pain, photophobia, and mid-dilated pupil
    d) rash, redness, and anterior chamber reaction

18. **If a patient has a localized allergic reaction to a topical medication instilled in the office, one should:**
    a) irrigate the eye immediately
    b) call 911
    c) administer oxygen, cortisone, and epinephrine
    d) check the pH of the eye and neutralize appropriately

19. **Abnormal drug reactions may occur:**
    a) in patients who are debilitated
    b) in the presence of other drugs
    c) as toxic or chemical reactions
    d) all of the above

20. **To prevent passage of a drug from the eye into the system as a whole and thereby decreasing the chances of systemic side effects, one should utilize:**
    a) medications that are cold
    b) medications that are room temperature
    c) more than one drop
    d) punctal occlusion

21. **Pupillary dilation, rapid pulse, increased respirations, and other "fight or flight" responses are generated by:**
    a) the voluntary nervous system
    b) the cranial nerves
    c) the parasympathetic system
    d) the sympathetic system

22. **The branch of the autonomic nervous system that is responsible for balancing the sympathetic system is the:**
    a) peripheral system
    b) parasympathetic system
    c) antisympathetic system
    d) adrenergic system

23. **The principal neurotransmitter(s) of the sympathetic nervous system is/are:**
    a) acetylcholine
    b) epinephrine (adrenaline) and norepinephrine
    c) cholinesterase
    d) insulin

24. **A cholinergic drug exerts its effect by impacting:**
    a) blood flow
    b) spinal nerves
    c) the sympathetic system
    d) the parasympathetic system

25. **A drug that copies the effect of the sympathetic system is known as:**
    a) sympathomimetic
    b) sympatholytic
    c) antagonistic
    d) cholinergic

26. **One example of a sympathomimetic drug is:**
    a) betaxolol
    b) dapiprazole
    c) pilocarpine
    d) phenylephrine

27. **The vasoconstrictors naphazoline and tetrahydrozoline fall into which group of drugs?**
    a) sympatholytic
    b) sympathomimetic
    c) parasympatholytic
    d) parasympathomimetic

28. **The glaucoma drugs apraclonidine and brimonidine are classified as:**
    a) sympathomimetic
    b) sympatholytic
    c) parasympathomimetic
    d) beta blockers

29. **A sympatholytic drug exerts its effect by:**
    a) inhibiting the parasympathetic pathway
    b) inhibiting cholinesterase
    c) enhancing the sympathetic pathway
    d) blocking the sympathetic pathway

30. **Timolol is an example of a:**
    a) parasympatholytic agent
    b) parasympathomimetic agent
    c) sympathomimetic agent
    d) sympatholytic agent

31. **Pupil dilation reversal via the topical drugs dapiprazole or thymoxamine is accomplished via:**
    a) enhancing the sympathetic system
    b) blocking of the sympathetic system
    c) destroying cholinesterase
    d) enhancing adrenaline

32. **An example of a parasympathomimetic drug is:**
    a) cocaine
    b) atropine
    c) pilocarpine
    d) carteolol

33. **The parasympathomimetics used in glaucoma treatment decrease IOP by means of:**
    a) increasing aqueous outflow
    b) decreasing aqueous production
    c) pupillary dilation
    d) increased blood flow to the eye

34. **An undesirable side effect of the miotics is brow ache, which is caused by the parasympathetic action of:**
    a) mydriasis
    b) iris sphincter contraction
    c) increased blood flow
    d) accommodative spasms

35. **A cholinergic-blocking drug (such as cyclopentolate) is an example of a(n):**
    a) parasympathomimetic drug
    b) parasympatholytic drug
    c) cholinesterase inhibitor
    d) sympatholytic drug

36. **An example of a parasympatholytic drug that is sometimes used to treat severe blepharospasm is:**
    a) edrophonium
    b) botulinum A toxin
    c) dapiprazole
    d) apraclonidine

37. **As a group, the following are parasympatholytic:**
    a) mydriatics
    b) cycloplegics
    c) miotics
    d) vasoconstrictors

38. **The biochemical cholinesterase acts on:**
    a) acetylcholine
    b) epinephrine
    c) norepinephrine
    d) aqueous

39. **Drugs that are cholinesterase inhibitors (anti-cholinesterases) will affect the:**
    a) levels of epinephrine
    b) voluntary nervous system
    c) sympathetic system
    d) parasympathetic system

40. As a group, the cholinesterase inhibitors include:
   a) the direct-acting miotics
   b) the indirect-acting miotics
   c) the beta blockers
   d) the cycloplegics

41. A cholinesterase inhibitor used in the differential diagnosis of ptosis is:
   a) cocaine
   b) edrophonium
   c) tetrahydrozoline
   d) botulinum A toxin

Chapter 9

Special Instruments and Techniques

Notes:

A-scan biometry is covered in *Certified Ophthalmic Assistant Exam Review Manual*.

Slit lamp illumination techniques are covered in this book under Chapter 7, Advanced Photography.

One category under this content area is "Macular Function Testing." There are many tests designed to measure macular function, including visual acuity, color vision, and contrast sensitivity. Since each of those tests have categories themselves, I judged that the macular photostress test and glare testing should be discussed here.

1. **A laser beam is created by exposing a chemical substance to a power source and amplification system in order to:**
   a) excite protons to emit polarized photons
   b) excite electrons to emit monochromatic photons
   c) excite neutrons to emit collimated photons
   d) slow down electrons to emit an intense photon stream

2. **The argon and krypton are examples of laser action via:**
   a) thermal photocoagulation
   b) ionizing (photodisruptive) reaction
   c) photochemical reaction
   d) photo-evaporation

3. **The argon laser is especially useful for procedures involving:**
   a) skin
   b) malignant tumors
   c) the macula
   d) blood vessels

4. **If the patient's IOP has been checked via Goldmann tonometry, before treatment with the argon laser, one should:**
   a) irrigate the fluorescein dye from the eye
   b) use a laser lens to bypass the tear film
   c) abort the procedure if the IOP is low
   d) proceed as usual

5. **The krypton laser might be used to:**
   a) trim sutures following trabeculectomy
   b) remove benign skin lesions
   c) remove malignant skin lesions
   d) lyse vitreous adhesions

6. **In comparison to the argon laser, the krypton laser is used to treat:**
   a) superficial blood vessels
   b) retinal blood vessels
   c) synechiae
   d) deep choroid, outer retina, and macula

7. **The ionizing YAG laser exerts its effect on tissues via:**
   a) thermal photocoagulation
   b) photodisruption
   c) photochemical reaction
   d) photoablation

8. **The YAG laser would likely be used for which of the following procedures?**
   a) treatment of diabetic retinopathy
   b) correcting refractive errors
   c) removal of skin lesions
   d) laser iridotomy

9. **The excimer laser utilizes a(n):**
   a) infrared wavelength
   b) ultraviolet wavelength
   c) adjustable wavelength
   d) blue-green wavelength

10. **The excimer laser has been approved for use in:**
    a) refractive surgery
    b) tumor treatment
    c) removal of skin cancers
    d) iridotomy

11. **The carbon dioxide laser is used to treat tissues that have a:**
    a) high melanin content
    b) high xanthophyll content
    c) high water content
    d) high hemoglobin content

12. **The carbon dioxide laser is used to:**
    a) sculpt the cornea in refractive surgery
    b) remove skin lesions and in eyelid surgery
    c) lyse vitreous adhesions
    d) perform iridotomies

13. **The advantage of tunable dye lasers is that:**
    a) various ultraviolet wavelengths can be selected
    b) various wavelengths from green to red can be selected
    c) various infrared wavelengths can be selected
    d) common fluorescein dye may be used

14. **The instrument used for internal cyclophotocoagulation is the:**
    a) cryolaser
    b) tunable dye laser
    c) laser microendoscope
    d) laser lathe

15. **Laser treatment involving a photochemical mechanism (laser interacting with a photo-sensitizing agent) has been used in ophthalmology to:**
    a) treat glaucoma
    b) remove tattoos
    c) treat cancerous growths
    d) reduce wrinkles

16. **The technology used in computerized tomography (CT) is based on using:**
    a) photography
    b) ionizing radiation
    c) magnetic radiation
    d) ultrasound

17. **Special dye may be injected as part of a CT study in order to:**
    a) help the patient relax
    b) trace blood flow in the tissues
    c) judge the reaction of the tissues to the dye
    d) provide contrast among the tissues

18. **The technology used in magnetic resonance imaging (MRI) is based on exposing the patient to:**
    a) ultrasonic waves
    b) radio waves
    c) ionizing radiation
    d) polarized light

19. **Which test would be most helpful in diagnosing an orbital fracture?**
    a) diagnostic B-scan
    b) MRI
    c) CT scan
    d) standardized A-scan

20. **A patient scheduled for an MRI gives a past medical history of having a pacemaker. This information is useful in order to:**
    a) cancel the MRI
    b) pre-medicate the patient
    c) notify the hospital not to use a microwave oven while the patient is there
    d) proceed as usual

21. **The physician suspects that the patient has a lesion in the chiasm. Which test would be most useful?**
    a) CT scan
    b) X-ray
    c) MRI
    d) B-scan ultrasound

22. **A two-dimensional image of the globe may be obtained by:**
    a) A-scan axial length ultrasonography
    b) diagnostic A-scan ultrasonography
    c) B-scan ultrasonography
    d) C-scan ultrasonography

23. **An example of a dynamic evaluation made during B-scan ultrasonography is:**
    a) measuring the dimensions of a tumor
    b) identifying highly reflective entities
    c) observing the after movement of a structure
    d) measuring the axial length

24. **During a B-scan, one observes quick, smooth movement of an apparent thin membrane. It is likely that the membrane is a(n):**
    a) vitreous detachment
    b) retinal detachment
    c) epiretinal membrane
    d) cloudy posterior capsule

25. **The patient has a dense traumatic cataract and count fingers vision with questionable pupillary response. The physician considering cataract surgery will often order a B-scan in this case in order to determine:**
    a) the patient's possible postoperative vision
    b) whether or not the retina is attached
    c) whether or not there is blood in the anterior chamber
    d) whether or not the eye is longer than normal

26. **Essentially, every ultrasonic device will have the following components:**
    a) gate, gain control, spike amplifier, and Ganzfeld bowl
    b) gas electron source, power source, and transmitter
    c) pulse emitter, receiver, amplifier, processor, and display
    d) ray emitter, crystal probe, monitor, and keyboard

27. **On an A- or B-scan, the gates or calipers refer to a:**
    a) wavelength
    b) spike height
    c) spike separation
    d) set of measurement markers

28. **The use of standardized A-scan in conjunction with a contact B-scan and standardized examination techniques is referred to as:**
    a) diagnostic ultrasonography
    b) standardized echography
    c) conditional echography
    d) real-time biometry

29. The top of the B-scan display screen corresponds to:
   a) the 12:00 position of the limbus
   b) the 12:00 position behind the equator
   c) the marker on the probe
   d) the position of the optic nerve in relation to the scan

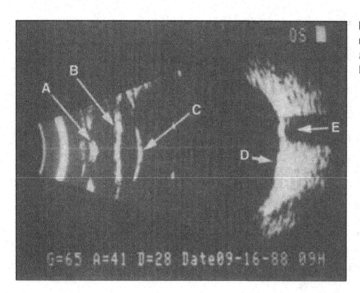

Figure 9-1. (Reprinted with permission from Kendall CJ. *Ophthalmic Echography*. Thorofare, NJ: SLACK Incorporated; 1990.)

30. Label the following on this B-scan (Figure 9-1):
   iris
   optic nerve
   cornea
   macula
   lens

31. Most artifacts in B-scan ultrasonography are caused by:
   a) poor contact between the probe and the eye
   b) improper gain settings
   c) glass intraocular foreign bodies
   d) intraocular air

32. In diagnostic B-scan, the position where the probe is placed on the cornea so that the optic nerve is in the center of the image is known as the:
   a) transverse view
   b) vertical axial view
   c) oblique view
   d) longitudinal view

33. On B-scan, you have detected an intraocular foreign body that is highly reflective and has a "shadow" behind it. Most likely, this foreign body is:
   a) plastic
   b) bone
   c) metal
   d) glass

Figure 9-2. (Reprinted with permission from Kendall CJ. *Ophthalmic Echography*. Thorofare, NJ: SLACK Incorporated; 1990.)

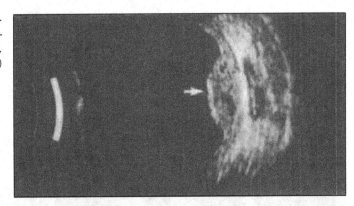

Figure 9-3. (Reprinted with permission from Kendall CJ. *Ophthalmic Echography*. Thorofare, NJ: SLACK Incorporated; 1990.)

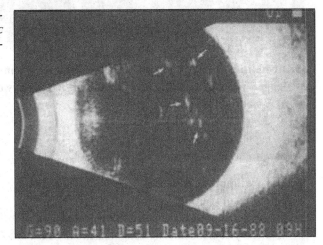

Figure 9-4. (Reprinted with permission from Kendall CJ. *Ophthalmic Echography*. Thorofare, NJ: SLACK Incorporated; 1990.)

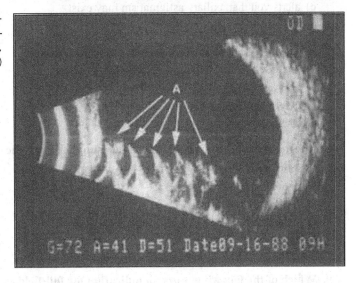

34. **Identify the entities shown in the following B-scans (Figures 9-2 through 9-5) as:**
    a) artifact
    b) intraocular tumor
    c) retinal detachment
    d) vitreous opacities

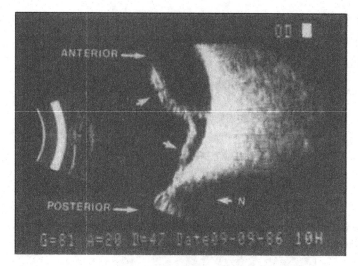

Figure 9-5. (Reprinted with permission from Kendall CJ. *Ophthalmic Echography*. Thorofare, NJ: SLACK Incorporated; 1990.)

35. **In addition to specifying the preoperative measurements of corneal curvature and axial length, when calculating intraocular lens (IOL) powers, one must also enter:**
    a) visible corneal diameter
    b) desired postoperative refractive error
    c) pupil size
    d) current refractive error

36. **You are inputting data for IOL calculations and notice that the K readings are 44.5/42.75. This type of reading:**
    a) should prompt you to repeat the measurement
    b) alerts you that lenticular astigmatism may exist
    c) alerts you that axillary astigmatism may exist
    d) is acceptable

37. **Almost all of the formulas for calculating IOL power:**
    a) are based on desiring emmetropia after surgery
    b) are based on measuring the aphakic eye
    c) are based on the same general equation
    d) are based on using an anterior chamber lens

38. **The manufacturer of a given IOL often supplies a specific number that must be entered into the IOL calculations when their lens is to be used. This number is referred to as a(n):**
    a) A-constant
    b) fudge factor
    c) personal identification number
    d) optical constant

39. **Which of the following is *not* an indication for full-field electroretinography (ERG)?**
    a) rule out the retina as the problem in suspected cortical blindness
    b) evaluate retinitis pigmentosa, night blindness, partial and total colorblindness
    c) evaluate macular degeneration and cortical blindness
    d) evaluate central retinal artery or vein occlusion, carotid insufficiency, drug toxicity

40. **The full-field electroretinogram (ERG) evaluates:**
    a) macular cone activity
    b) both rod and cone activity
    c) rod activity only
    d) cone activity only

41. **If the amplitude of the ERG results is reduced by 50%, this indicates that:**
    a) 50% of the retina is not functioning
    b) 50% of the macula is not functioning
    c) the retina takes twice as long to respond to the stimulus
    d) this can only be ascertained with a computer program

42. **The electrodes used in ERG testing are:**
    a) active and ground
    b) stationary and mobile
    c) active, reference, and ground
    d) static and kinetic

43. **Before beginning the ERG, the patient is:**
    a) light-adapted
    b) dark-adapted
    c) dilated and light-adapted
    d) dilated and dark-adapted

44. **A flicker fusion ERG may be contraindicated in a patient with a history of:**
    a) angina
    b) epilepsy
    c) diabetes
    d) anxiety

45. **The protocol for ERG evaluation includes:**
    a) pattern, sinusoidal, and object targets
    b) scotopic, mesopic, oscillatory potential, photopic, and flicker fusion
    c) subjective responses by the patient
    d) dilated and undilated evaluations

46. **The ERG waveform is composed of:**
    a) an a-wave created by the Mueller and bipolar cells and a b-wave generated by the photo-receptor cells
    b) an a-wave created by the photoreceptor cells and a b-wave generated by the Mueller and bipolar cells
    c) an a-wave generated by the rods and a b-wave generated by the cones
    d) an a-wave generated by the cones and a b-wave generated by the rods

47. **The ERG of a patient with end-stage retinitis pigmentosa would likely show:**
    a) slowing of the waves
    b) a reduction in amplitude of both a- and b-waves
    c) normal a-waves and abnormal b-waves
    d) a non-recordable ERG

48. The purpose of the electrooculograph (EOG) is to evaluate the function of the:
   a) rods
   b) cones
   c) retinal pigment epithelium
   d) retina as a whole

49. The read-outs generated during the EOG are the result of:
   a) eye movements only
   b) eye movements and electrical changes across the eye between the retina and cornea
   c) eye movements and electrical changes between the rods and the cones
   d) eye movements and electrical changes between the macula and peripheral retina

50. Patient preparation for an EOG includes:
   a) dilation, a corneal and skin electrode, and dark-adaptation
   b) best corrected visual acuity and light-adaptation
   c) three to 12 skin electrodes and dark- followed by light-adaptation
   d) dilation, five skin electrodes, and light- followed by dark-adaptation

51. In evaluating retinal function with the EOG, the eye movements are used to calculate a(n):
   a) A-constant
   b) Arden ratio
   c) overall retinal voltage factor
   d) mass retinal response

52. The Arden ratio in a patient with end-stage retinitis pigmentosa would be:
   a) 4.00
   b) 2.00
   c) 1.20
   d) 95%

53. Disorders where a retinal EOG might be useful include:
   a) retinal detachment, central retinal artery or vein occlusion, carotid artery insufficiency
   b) retinitis pigmentosa, Best's disease, retinal toxicities
   c) identification of malingering patient, evaluation of cortical blindness
   d) nystagmus, nerve palsies

54. When eliciting eye movements with the EOG to evaluate extraocular muscle function:
   a) the alternating diodes are used
   b) an optokinetic drum is used
   c) no electrodes are needed
   d) extraocular muscle function cannot be evaluated with the EOG

55. Indications for an EOG to evaluate eye movements include:
   a) nerve palsies and mechanical restrictions
   b) differentiate between a phoria and tropia
   c) cases of monocular diplopia
   d) none of the above

56. **The visually evoked potential (VEP) is an evaluation of the response to a visual stimulus by the:**
    a) cornea
    b) sclera
    c) occipital cortex
    d) extraocular muscles

57. **The stimulus(i) most used in the VEP testing is:**
    a) a set of sinusoidal gratings
    b) optotypes
    c) horizontal and vertical rotating bars
    d) flashing light and alternating checkerboard pattern

58. **Patient preparation for VEP testing includes:**
    a) attaching 3 to 12 scalp electrodes, occluding the untested eye
    b) dilation, a corneal electrode and scalp electrode, dark adaptation
    c) fogging the non-tested eye with +6.00 sphere, 3 to 12 scalp electrodes
    d) topical ocular anesthetic, a corneal electrode, occlusion of untested eye

59. **If the patient fails to respond to the largest VEP checkerboard pattern:**
    a) visual acuity may be worse than 20/400
    b) he or she has a normal visual system and 20/20 acuity
    c) try again with a smaller pattern
    d) this is a normal response

60. **The indications for VEP testing include:**
    a) macular degeneration, retinal detachment
    b) media opacity
    c) unexplained vision loss, evaluating visual potential
    d) determining the cause of blindness

61. **The waveform generated by the flash VEP is:**
    a) weak at first, then gets stronger
    b) a wave of a single peak
    c) indistinguishable from other brain activity
    d) complex, with positive peaks (labeled P) and negative peaks (labeled N)

62. **Dark adaptometry is a subjective test which primarily evaluates:**
    a) how long it takes for the retina to recover from being light-bleached
    b) the degree to which the rods become increasingly sensitive in the dark
    c) how quickly the pupils respond to dim-light conditions
    d) the degree to which the cones become increasingly sensitive in the dark

63. **Disorders that can be evaluated by dark adaptometry include:**
    a) only rod disorders
    b) only cone disorders
    c) both rod and cone disorders
    d) identification of malingering patients

64. **Before the dark-adapting phase of dark adaptometry begins, the patient is:**
    a) dilated
    b) photographed
    c) light-adapted
    d) fully dark-adapted

65. **During the dark-adapting phase of dark adaptometry:**
    a) the cones are tested for the first 5 minutes, and then the rods are tested for the remaining 25 minutes
    b) the rods are tested for the first 30 minutes, and then the cones are tested
    c) only the rods are tested, since cones are not sensitive in the dark
    d) the retinal periphery is tested for the first 30 minutes, and then the macula is tested

66. **In dark adaptometry, the rod-cone break is represented by:**
    a) the continued dark adaptation of the cones over time
    b) the rising of the cone curve and declining of the rod curve
    c) the crossing of the cone and rod curves
    d) the declining of the cone curve and the rising of the rod curve

67. **In a patient with retinitis pigmentosa or other rod dysfunction, the results of dark adaptometry will show:**
    a) no response of any kind
    b) an abnormal cone response but a normal rod curve
    c) both curves are normal
    d) the cone response is normal but there is no rod curve

68. **In order to determine how quickly a patient's vision returns to near-normal after being exposed to a bright light, one might perform the:**
    a) glare test
    b) macular photostress test
    c) dark adaptometry
    d) direct pupil exam

69. **When being evaluated by the macular photostress test, the recovery time for a normal macula should be less than:**
    a) 10 seconds
    b) 20 seconds
    c) 50 seconds
    d) 90 seconds

70. **The Potential Acuity Meter (Marco Technologies Inc, Jacksonville, Fla) is commonly used to evaluate macular function in the presence of:**
    a) glaucoma
    b) retinal disorders
    c) optic nerve disease
    d) media opacities

71. **Before performing a Potential Acuity Meter test, it is important to:**
    a) set the eyepiece
    b) enter the patient's refractive error
    c) calibrate the unit
    d) have the patient wear his or her best correction

72. **Pupillography involves photographing the pupil by using:**
    a) a ring flash
    b) infrared lighting
    c) ultraviolet lighting
    d) laser-enhanced lighting

73. **Which of the following conditions apply during pupillography?**
    a) a dilated pupil
    b) an undilated pupil
    c) fluorescein dye is used
    d) ICG dye is used

74. **In pupillography, both eyes are filmed simultaneously as the direct and consensual responses are elicited. The results are then:**
    a) viewed directly
    b) transferred to a graph
    c) evaluated using a grid overlay
    d) recorded simultaneously on a revolving drum

75. **For the widest field of view when examining the fundus, one would use the:**
    a) Hruby lens
    b) indirect ophthalmoscope
    c) direct ophthalmoscope
    d) minus contact lens and the slit lamp

76. **Using the green filter on the direct ophthalmoscope is most useful when examining:**
    a) the macula
    b) the vitreous
    c) blood vessels and retinal nerve fibers
    d) structures anterior to the equator

77. **The slit beam available in the direct ophthalmoscope would be used when evaluating:**
    a) retinal lesions
    b) optic disc cupping
    c) nicking in the blood vessels
    d) the vitreous

78. **When evaluating the fundus using the indirect ophthalmoscope, a view of structures anterior to the equator may be seen:**
    a) in stereo
    b) if scleral depression is utilized
    c) using a contact mirrored lens
    d) none of the above

79. **Factors related to indirect ophthalmoscopy include:**
    a) no need to dilate the pupil
    b) an up-right image
    c) compensation for the patient's refractive error
    d) none of the above

80. **Items that are evaluated during ophthalmoscopy include:**
    a) tear film, corneal clarity, refractive error
    b) accommodation, pupillary reflex, anterior chamber reaction
    c) media clarity, fundus reflex, cup-to-disc ratio
    d) none of the above

81. **The feature(s) that has made the slit lamp biomicroscope ideal for ocular examination is:**
    a) the optical section
    b) variable magnifications
    c) various filters
    d) binocularity

82. **When beginning the slit lamp exam, it is *least* advantageous to set the magnification on:**
    a) 6X
    b) 10X
    c) 16X
    d) 40X

83. **Which of the following would be the correct way to document a slit lamp finding?**
    a) WNL
    b) 3+ blepharitis
    c) 2+ lash crusting with 3+ lid edema
    d) 4+ viral conjunctivitis

84. **When evaluating anterior chamber depth, the illumination technique used is:**
    a) diffuse
    b) direct, narrow beam
    c) direct, wide beam
    d) proximal

85. **When evaluating the fit of a rigid contact lens using the slit lamp and fluorescein dye, in addition to the cobalt blue light, contrast can be improved by using a:**
    a) red-free filter
    b) green filter
    c) Wratten filter
    d) diffuser

86. **The slit lamp may be used to evaluate the posterior pole if one uses a(n):**
    a) ophthalmoscope
    b) cross-hair reticule
    c) scleral depressor
    d) Hruby lens

87. **The design of the photokeratoscope is based on the:**
    a) keratometer
    b) Placido's disk
    c) slit lamp
    d) specular microscope

88. **The most common artifact present on photokeratoscopy is caused by:**
    a) the camera flash
    b) a dry cornea
    c) the patient's refractive error
    d) an unfocused eyepiece

89. **True corneal irregularities may be documented with the photokeratoscope if:**
    a) alignment and focus are accurate
    b) the patient's refractive error is neutralized
    c) the patient is wearing a soft contact lens
    d) there is no pooling of fluorescein dye

90. **In photokeratoscopy of a flat cornea, the spacing of the rings will:**
    a) be broken in the same area
    b) vary
    c) be farther apart
    d) be closer together

Figure 9-6. (Reprinted with permission from Van Boemel GB. *Special Skills and Techniques.* Thorofare, NJ: SLACK Incorporated; 1999.)

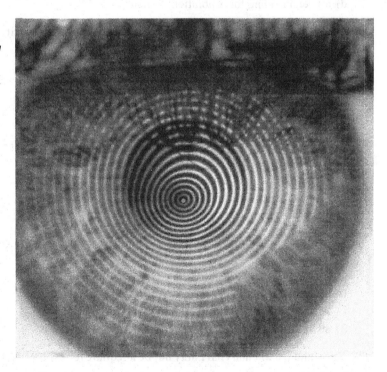

91. **In this photokeratoscopy (Figure 9-6), the condition illustrated is:**
    a) corneal astigmatism; steeper inferiorly
    b) corneal astigmatism; steeper superiorly
    c) mixed corneal astigmatism
    d) emmetropia

92. **Measuring corneal thickness via non-optical pachymetry involves the use of:**
    a) specular microscopy
    b) ultrasound
    c) the slit lamp microscope
    d) a contact mirrored lens

93. **One of the keys in accurate pachymetry is:**
    a) aiming the probe at the optic nerve
    b) aiming the probe at the macula
    c) maintaining contact with the coupling gel
    d) holding the probe perpendicular to the corneal surface

94. **Pachymetry readings are routinely taken prior to:**
    a) cataract surgery
    b) retinal surgery
    c) refractive surgery
    d) plastic surgery

95. **When performing pachymetry, it is generally best to begin:**
    a) with the corneal periphery at 12:00
    b) with the central cornea
    c) with the mid-periphery at 12:00
    d) a scleral reading for calibration

96. **Which of the following is *not* true regarding distant visual acuity charts designed specifically for testing low vision patients?**
    a) it provides lower contrast
    b) it provides larger optotypes than traditional charts
    c) it provides more graded lines in the larger sizes
    d) it provides continuous reading text

97. **When testing near vision in the low vision patient, the best type of card to use is the:**
    a) continuous text
    b) same chart used for distance
    c) contrast sensitivity card
    d) any near chart may be used

98. **In addition to testing visual acuity of the low vision patient, it is also advantageous to perform:**
    a) contrast sensitivity testing
    b) glare testing
    c) Amsler grid
    d) all of the above

99. **The standard Snellen chart may not be adequate for evaluating how a patient really sees because:**
    a) it cannot be used in varying light conditions
    b) it does not measure macular function
    c) it is high contrast
    d) it is easy to memorize

100. **The test objects used in contrast sensitivity testing all use:**
    a) graduated contrast
    b) Snellen equivalents
    c) laser-enhanced graphics
    d) various lighting conditions

101. **When testing the patient's contrast sensitivity, the following correction should be used:**
    a) none
    b) patient's habitual correction
    c) best correction
    d) spherical equivalent

102. **During contrast sensitivity testing, it is important that the patient:**
    a) be urged to guess even when not sure
    b) respond only when definitely sure of the answer
    c) maintain alignment
    d) stop when unsure of the answer

103. **During contrast sensitivity testing using sinusoidal gratings, the score sheet is marked to indicate the last correctly identified object in each row. This information is used to:**
    a) calculate potential acuity
    b) plot a contrast sensitivity curve
    c) calculate vision loss due to media opacities
    d) determine disability ratings

104. **At this time it is not possible to differentiate ocular disease on the basis of contrast sensitivity alone because:**
    a) there has not been adequate research
    b) ocular disorders do not have specific contrast abnormalities
    c) frequency losses tend to overlap
    d) the test is not standardized

Chapter 10

Advanced General Medical Knowledge

1. **The retinal blood vessels of diabetics sometimes develop bulges known as:**
   a) emboli
   b) microaneurysms
   c) artheromas
   d) exudates

2. **Blindness in diabetics is mainly caused by:**
   a) microaneurysms
   b) macular edema
   c) optic nerve damage
   d) elevated IOP

3. **In diabetics, the small retinal vessels may become blocked, depriving the retina of oxygen. The body's response to this situation is:**
   a) neovascularization
   b) atrophy
   c) hemorrhage
   d) edema

4. **The difference between background and proliferative diabetic retinopathy is that proliferative retinopathy exhibits:**
   a) no appreciable worsening
   b) only cotton wool spots
   c) only soft exudates
   d) neovascularization and venous bleeding

5. **The occurrence of diabetic retinopathy is mainly related to:**
   a) the type of medication used to control it
   b) whether or not the patient is obese
   c) the duration of the diabetes
   d) the presence or absence of other eye disease

6. **Other ocular problems seen in diabetics include:**
   a) recurrent infections
   b) early onset of presbyopia
   c) cataracts, refractive fluctuations, and muscle palsies
   d) optic neuropathy, nystagmus, and diplopia

7. **On ophthalmoscopic evaluation of a patient with hypertension, you notice that the walls of the vessels have an odd reflex, appearing copper or silver colored. This is caused by:**
   a) fibrous tissue lining the vessel walls
   b) fatty tissue lining the vessel walls
   c) emboli
   d) light refraction by a hypertensive cataract

8. **In the more advanced stages of hypertensive retinopathy, changes in the retinal vessels include:**
   a) neovascularization
   b) straightening and/or twisting of the vessels
   c) development of shunt vessels
   d) microaneurysms

9. **Serious visual impairment in the patient with hypertensive retinopathy most often occurs as the result of:**
   a) associated cataracts
   b) associated retinal scarring
   c) artery or vein occlusions
   d) retinal detachment

10. **The key in treating hypertensive retinopathy seems to be:**
    a) type of medication used to control the pressure
    b) duration of the disorder
    c) blood pressure control
    d) whether or not glaucoma develops as a complication

11. **The most common effect of atherosclerosis on the eye is:**
    a) artery obstruction
    b) hemorrhage
    c) traction retinal detachment
    d) formation of microaneurysms

12. **The main cause of unilateral or bilateral exophthalmus in adults is:**
    a) pseudotumor
    b) neuroblastoma
    c) Graves' disease
    d) orbital cellulitis

13. **The ocular changes seen in Graves' disease are mainly due to:**
    a) lack of blood supply
    b) involvement of the extraocular muscles
    c) macular edema
    d) associated uveitis

14. **Early signs of ophthalmic Graves' disease are:**
    a) lid retraction, lid lag, intermittent stare
    b) cotton wool spots and exudates
    c) opacified deposits in the cornea and lens
    d) central scotomata, metamorphopsia, and fluctuating refractive error

15. **Vision loss in Graves' disease can be due to:**
    a) elevated IOP and optic nerve damage
    b) media opacities
    c) rapid rotary nystagmus
    d) corneal dryness or optic nerve compression

16. **Diplopia in patients with Graves' ophthalmopathy is due to:**
    a) fibrosis of the muscles
    b) adhesions between the muscles
    c) compression of the muscles
    d) any of the above

17. **The patient with low thyroid levels (hypothyroid or myxedema) may exhibit:**
    a) keratoconus, mild cataracts, and optic atrophy
    b) elevated IOP and narrow angles
    c) tortuous retinal blood vessels
    d) chronic blepharitis, trichiasis, and corneal scarring

18. **Pituitary tumors generally affect the:**
    a) retina
    b) optic nerve
    c) optic chiasm
    d) visual cortex

19. **The visual field defect generally seen in pituitary tumor is:**
    a) binasal hemianopsia
    b) loss of both right fields
    c) bitemporal hemianopsia
    d) loss of both left fields

20. **If the pressure on the chiasm due to a pituitary tumor is not relieved, the following can occur:**
    a) optic nerve atrophy and permanent vision loss
    b) narrowing of the anterior chamber and angle closure attacks
    c) amaurosis fugax
    d) death

21. **If a pituitary tumor secretes large amounts of hormones, this could cause:**
    a) Sturge-Weber syndrome
    b) Cushing's syndrome
    c) Down syndrome
    d) Tay-Sachs disease

22. **The symptoms caused by brain tumors are often related to:**
    a) increased intracranial pressure
    b) metastases to the orbit
    c) metastases to the uvea
    d) interruptions to ocular blood flow

23. **Symptoms of brain tumor can include:**
    a) floaters, flashes, curtain over vision
    b) decreased vision, nausea and vomiting, halos around lights
    c) optic nerve cupping, retinal hemorrhage, elevated IOP
    d) headache, diplopia, decreased vision, nausea and vomiting

24. **In addition to visual field defects, a tumor of the occipital lobe may be associated with:**
    a) disturbances in color vision
    b) a decrease in the eye's axial length
    c) disturbances of pursuit movements and nystagmus
    d) poor dark adaptation

25. **Amaurosis fugax is mainly associated with:**
    a) vascular disease
    b) neoplasms
    c) muscular disorders
    d) neurological disorders

26. **A patient presents with unilateral keratoconjunctivitis, a painful rash on one side of the face, and a history of chicken pox infection as a child. It is very likely that this patient has:**
    a) Herpes simplex
    b) Herpes zoster
    c) rubella
    d) contact dermatitis

27. **The most common ocular findings in patients with acquired immunodeficiency syndrome (AIDS) are:**
    a) retinal scarring
    b) keratoconjunctivitis
    c) changes in retinal and conjunctival blood vessels
    d) ocular infections

28. **The triad of xerostomia (dry mouth), keratoconjunctivitis sicca, and connective tissue disease (usually rheumatoid arthritis) are known as:**
    a) rheumatoid eye
    b) xerophthalmia
    c) Graves' disease
    d) Sjogren's syndrome

29. **The most serious ocular effects of malnutrition are due to the lack of:**
    a) vitamin A
    b) vitamin C
    c) zinc
    d) vitamin E

30. **The most common ocular problem associated with smoking is:**
    a) increased risk of nuclear sclerotic cataract
    b) increased risk of macular degeneration
    c) more severe optic nerve damage in glaucoma patients
    d) chronic conjunctival irritation

31. **Ocular findings associated with gout include:**
    a) under-active extraocular muscles
    b) elevated IOP and injection
    c) recurrent infections
    d) nystagmus

32. **Multiple sclerosis, in which the myelin sheath of the nerves breaks down, is often manifest in the eye by:**
    a) optic neuritis
    b) leukocoria
    c) optic cupping
    d) fluctuating vision

33. **In patients with myasthenia gravis, the symptoms of lid droop and diplopia are caused by:**
    a) poor nerve connections
    b) muscle fatigue
    c) poor patient cooperation
    d) poor blood supply to the extraocular muscles

34. **The connective tissue disease marked by elongation of the long bones and lens dislocation is:**
    a) rheumatoid arthritis
    b) systemic lupus erythematosus
    c) Marfan's syndrome
    d) sarcoidosis

35. **Glaucoma associated with asthma, emphysema, and rheumatoid arthritis is most often due to:**
    a) use of systemic steroids
    b) narrowing of the anterior chamber
    c) a change in the diurnal curve
    d) connective tissue damage

36. **The term "legal blindness" refers to which best corrected acuity (in the better eye) or which limitation of peripheral vision?**
    a) 20/40 and 60 degrees
    b) 20/100 and 40 degrees
    c) 20/200 and 20 degrees
    d) 20/400 and 20 degrees

37. **Your patient's best corrected acuity in the better eye is 20/100. Because he does not qualify as legally blind:**
    a) he is not eligible for any type of assistance
    b) he cannot be referred to a low vision clinic
    c) he may still be disabled and eligible for some type of compensation
    d) no optical low vision aids will be helpful

38. **When considering the degree of visual disability, the following factor(s) may be taken into account:**
    a) contrast sensitivity and glare
    b) binocular pseudophakia
    c) media opacities
    d) monocular aphakia or pseudophakia

39. **The largest group of individuals who are legally blind are:**
    a) preschool children (infants to age 5)
    b) school-aged children (ages 5 to 18)
    c) young adults
    d) elderly persons

40. **The leading cause of blindness in adults living in the Western world is:**
    a) cataracts
    b) glaucoma
    c) retinal disease
    d) trachoma

41. **Which of the following is true regarding cortical blindness?**
    a) the patient has normal pupils, clear media, and a normal-appearing fundus
    b) it occurs in the visual pathway at some point beyond the geniculate body
    c) it can be associated with stroke, multiple sclerosis, and brain tumor
    d) all of the above

42. **Of those who are legally blind:**
    a) most have some residual vision
    b) most are totally blind
    c) most have developed nystagmus
    d) most have tunnel vision

43. **Rehabilitation for the totally blind might include:**
    a) physical therapy and referral to social services
    b) annual eye exams and eye motility exercises
    c) non-optical aids, mobility training, and psychological counseling
    d) optical aids, vocational rehabilitation, and physical therapy

44. **Determining the functional vision of the legally blind patient may include:**
    a) glare testing
    b) visual acuity and contrast sensitivity
    c) visual fields
    d) all of the above

45. **In order to *best* assess the legally blind patient's functional vision at near, one should:**
    a) encourage the patient to guess at the letters on the acuity chart
    b) simply ask if the patient can see that there are letters on the chart; reading them is not necessary
    c) have the patient read only the smallest text that can be read easily and comfortably
    d) try all available low vision aids until finding the one that gives the best acuity

46. Visual efficiency is a product of:
a) loss of central acuity and peripheral field
b) loss of ocular motility and stereopsis
c) loss of binocular vision and peripheral field
d) areas where the vision is diplopic

47. Patients who are experiencing low vision for the first time:
a) generally adjust quickly if the family is supportive
b) should be put into rehabilitation immediately
c) will experience periods of sadness, fear, and grief
d) should be given hope that the condition will improve

48. Mrs. Smith has macular degeneration. She confides in you that she is now afraid to read anymore for fear of losing the remaining vision she has. You can tell her:
a) that is a good idea
b) using her eyes will not harm them
c) using her eyes will strengthen them
d) nothing; it is not the place of the technologist to discuss this

49. Patients with new-onset low vision or blindness often find:
a) that their other senses are sharpened
b) that it is very easy to remain useful and independent
c) that they must find new ways to relax and relieve stress
d) that they are still regarded as "part of the group"

50. The needs of a low vision patient are best determined by:
a) careful refractometry
b) showing him or her various types of aids
c) a careful history
d) agencies who assist the visually impaired

51. Your patient is a 4-year-old who has been blind since birth. During the exam, you observe that she repeatedly pushes on her eyes with her thumbs, and rocks in the chair. These mannerisms are known as:
a) rhythmic patterns
b) autism
c) blindisms
d) Oedipus syndrome

52. Which of the following is *not* true regarding trachoma?
a) it is associated with poor hygiene in Third World countries
b) findings include follicles, conjunctival scarring, corneal pannus, and corneal scarring
c) it is difficult to treat
d) it is caused by *Chlamydia trachomatis*

53. Which of the following is the most common proven cause of chorioretinitis?
a) toxoplasmosis
b) histoplasmosis
c) trachoma
d) trauma

54. Which of the following is *not* true of epidemic keratoconjunctivitis (EKC)?
    a) it is also called shipyard eye
    b) it is caused by the adenovirus
    c) it may be accompanied by lid swelling and conjunctival petechia
    d) it may be accompanied by a general malaise

55. **Orbital cellulitis usually occurs as the result of:**
    a) infection associated with trauma
    b) spread of bacteria from contaminated surfaces
    c) spread of infection from the ethmoid sinuses
    d) spread of infection from the meninges

56. **The patient has a severely injured eye with no hope of recovery. The physician has recommended an enucleation. This recommendation is based on the concern that:**
    a) a prosthesis will be more cosmetically appealing than the injured globe
    b) endophthalmitis may develop
    c) sympathetic ophthalmia may develop
    d) secondary glaucoma may develop

57. **Which of the following is *not* true regarding endophthalmitis?**
    a) the most common type of occurrence is following ocular trauma
    b) it involves vitreous abscess and inflammation of the intraocular tissues
    c) it is more commonly seen in immunocompromised individuals
    d) it occurs in part because the vitreous is an excellent culture medium

58. **Which one of the following corneal entities is caused by allergies or chemical toxicity?**
    a) guttata
    b) infectious infiltrates
    c) sterile infiltrates
    d) Krukenberg's spindle

59. **Which of the following is *not* true regarding vernal conjunctivitis?**
    a) it is seasonal, occurring during the cold months
    b) it produces enlarged papillae under the upper lid
    c) the patient may complain of a foreign body sensation, itching, and tearing
    d) it is basically an allergic response

60. **A coloboma is a congenital defect classified as:**
    a) a developmental/fusion defect
    b) a genetic defect
    c) a tissue reaction to intrauterine insult
    d) a developmental defect due to tissue overgrowth

61. **Retinopathy of prematurity (ROP), previously called retrolental fibroplasia (RLF), occurs when normal retinal vascular growth is interrupted, mainly due to:**
    a) early exposure to light
    b) lack of oxygen
    c) oxygen toxicity
    d) artificial ventilation

62. Which of the following is *not* true regarding albinism?
    a) it may present as strictly an ocular condition or as a condition involving both the skin and eye
    b) the patient generally has a problem with photophobia
    c) the patient generally has poor vision and nystagmus
    d) the patient always has pink skin and white hair

63. The most common type of vascular tumor seen in the newborn or small child is a:
    a) capillary hemangioma (strawberry nevus)
    b) port wine stain
    c) dermoid cyst
    d) retinoblastoma

64. Which of the following is *not* a malignant eyelid tumor?
    a) basal cell carcinoma
    b) squamous cell carcinoma
    c) melanoma
    d) papilloma

65. This type of malignancy can occur on the lids and conjunctiva. If it occurs intraocularly, however, it is limited to the uveal tract and may be associated with secondary glaucoma.
    a) squamous cell carcinoma
    b) melanoma
    c) basal cell carcinoma
    d) molluscum contagiosum

66. Which of the following is *not* one of the danger signals that a cutaneous nevus may be cancerous or potentially cancerous?
    a) irregular shape and border
    b) change in color
    c) dimpled center, bleeds and does not heal
    d) raised surface

67. Which of the following is a congenital tumor of the photoreceptors that is generally diagnosed by age 3?
    a) retinitis pigmentosa
    b) leukocoria
    c) retinoblastoma
    d) intraocular dermoid

68. This type of corneal dystrophy may progress to the point where bullous keratopathy and edema occur. Vision gradually decreases as the disorder progresses. Women are affected more than men. Initial treatment may include topical hypertonic sodium chloride.
    a) fingerprint dystrophy
    b) map-dot dystrophy
    c) ectatic dystrophy
    d) Fuch's dystrophy

69. **Cystoid macular edema is most commonly associated with:**
    a) trauma
    b) intraocular surgery
    c) angle-closure glaucoma
    d) wet (exudative) macular degeneration

70. **A degenerative process involving the vitreous in which the gel shrinks (usually with age) is:**
    a) asteroid hyalosis
    b) syneresis
    c) posterior vitreous detachment
    d) vitreous collapse

71. **In trauma where there is suspected corneal perforation with leakage of aqueous, the following test might be done to confirm this:**
    a) Schirmer's test
    b) Seidel's test
    c) Tensilon test
    d) Cole/Meeks test

72. **An injury in which the trauma is caused, not by direct contact but rather by the conduction of force through the tissues, is known as a:**
    a) laceration
    b) contusion
    c) concussion
    d) radiation

73. **Your patient was in a motor vehicle accident in which the force of impact momentarily pushed the iris onto the anterior lens surface. On slit lamp examination, this occurrence is evident by the presence of:**
    a) a traumatic cataract
    b) Vossius' ring
    c) posterior synechiae
    d) anterior synechiae

74. **Your patient has a history of being struck in the eye with high-velocity iron particles approximately 9 months ago. At that time, his vision was 20/25 and several foreign bodies were removed from the cornea, conjunctiva, and lids. His vision is now 20/70 and he complains that the iris is changing color. His IOP in that eye is 28 mmHg (12 mmHg in the other eye). This description suggests that the patient may have:**
    a) Crouzon's disease
    b) ghost cell glaucoma
    c) sarcoidosis
    d) siderosis

75. Your patient reports a foreign body sensation and decreased vision in one eye following an explosion in a lab in which shattered plastic became air-born. No chemicals were involved. Although she is not in a great deal of discomfort, you note the following: VA 20/80, D-shaped pupil, small area of brown exudate on the sclera at 9:00. These findings lead you to suspect a(n):
    a) perforated globe
    b) bacterial contamination
    c) embedded scleral foreign body
    d) traumatic scleral tattoo

76. A patient phones the office stating that his eyelid has just been cut by barbed wire. "It's only a little half-inch cut," he says. When he reports that the laceration is in the nasal canthus area of his lower lid, you recommend he be seen immediately. A possible complication of poor healing in this case could lead to a chronic problem with:
    a) entropion
    b) trichiasis
    c) dry eye
    d) epiphora

77. Your patient has a blow-out fracture. The eye has receded and dropped somewhat down into the maxillary sinus cavity. This situation is known as:
    a) anophthalmus
    b) microphthalmus
    c) enophthalmus
    d) retroglobus

78. Your patient has come in for a routine eye exam. Past ocular history (for which you happen to have records) includes a blunt trauma to the right eye 5 years ago which involved a 50% hyphema. She has had normal annual exams since that time. Today the patient has no complaints and all visual screening is normal. However, when you check her IOP, your readings are 27 mmHg in the right eye and 16 mmHg in the left. Gonioscopy of the right eye shows a large area where the insertion of the iris is more posterior than normal. This scenario describes:
    a) ghost cell glaucoma
    b) angle-recession glaucoma
    c) epithelial in-growth
    d) hemolytic glaucoma

79. Your patient was hit temporally in the left eye area with a tennis ball an hour ago. The eye is not yet swollen shut. On confrontation visual fields, there is a loss of field on the temporal side of the left eye. The right eye is normal. The physician notes retinal swelling nasally and a grayish-white opacification at the macula, but normal blood flow through the retinal vessels. This scenario describes:
    a) commotio retinae
    b) choroidal rupture
    c) cystoid macular edema
    d) epiretinal membrane

Chapter 11

Explanatory Answers

Chapter 1. Microbiology

1. b) The classic signs of inflammation, as identified in the first century and basically unchanged since that time, are redness, swelling, warmth (fever), and pain. These are associated with vascular changes. Chemical mediators, released when tissue injury occurs, cause vasodilation (Figure 11-1). The increased blood causes redness and warmth. The dilated vessels permit fluid to leak, causing swelling. The swelling puts pressure on local nerve endings, causing pain.

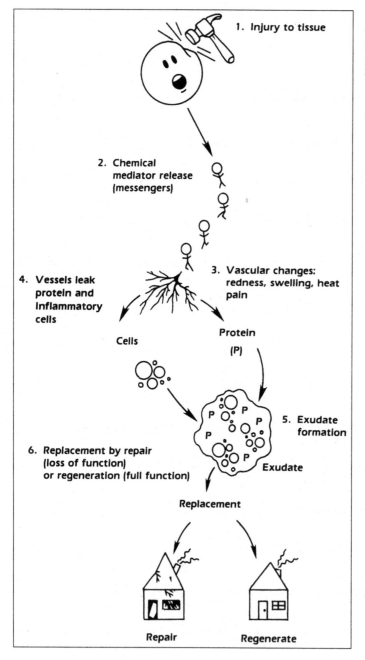

Figure 11-1. Schematic showing the inflammatory process. (Reprinted with permission from Nemeth SC, Shea CA. *Medical Sciences for the Ophthalmic Assistant.* Thorofare, NJ: SLACK Incorporated; 1988.)

2. a) The chemical mediators are released when tissue damage occurs. There are many such mediators, but the most important include histamine, prostaglandins, seratonin, kinins, and complement.

3. b) Antibodies (also known as immunoglobulins) are produced by the body in response to antigens (particles that the body recognizes as "non-self"). The spleen and lymph nodes are the primary sites of production.

4. d) First, an antigen stimulates formation of antibodies. The antibodies bind to the antigen. Complement is a substance (found in serum and plasma cells) that binds to an antibody. It destroys the cell wall to which the antibody is attached. If the antibody is attached to a bacterium, the complement ruptures the bacterial cell wall, destroying the cell.

5. d) Bacteria (including *Pseudomonas aeruginosa*), viruses (including *Herpes*), *Chlamydia* (with characteristics of viruses and bacteria), fungi (including *Candida albicans*), and protozoa (including *Toxocara canis* and *Acanthameobae*) are all infectious agents capable of causing ocular inflammation.

6. d) A highly virulent pathogen (organism capable of causing disease) would be extremely toxic or poisonous to the host.

7. d) A pathogen can cause an inflammatory response due to toxins (substances that are poisonous to the host, such as waste products), enzymes (substances that enhance the pathogen's survival by destruction of host materials), replication (taking over the host's cells or tissues for reproduction of the pathogen), or allergic reaction to toxins.

8. a) The inflammatory response can also be caused by non-infectious events such as trauma, inheritance (genetic disorders), autoimmunity (in which the body attacks its own cells), and nutritional deficiencies (lack of substances needed to keep the body healthy).

9. a) Inflammatory cells cause various entities depending on the tissue where they manifest. Papillae (palpebral conjunctiva), infiltrates (cornea), hypopyon (white cells in the anterior chamber), and exudates (retina) are all examples. Others are follicles (palpebral conjunctiva), cells (anterior chamber), purulent discharge, and mucus discharge.

10. d) A granulocyte is a mature white blood cell that contains granules. The type of granulocyte is determined by the type of granules that the cell contains.

See Table 11-1 for Explanations of Questions 11 through 16.

11. b)

12. a)

13. a)

14. b)

15. d)

16. a)

Table 11-1
In ammatory Cells

Neutrophile (also called polymorphonucleocyte, poly, or PMN)

Appearance: Multi-lobed nucleus with pink cytoplasm.
Function: They are the first line of defense in inflammation. They release enzymes and eat bacteria and are seen in any case of inflammation, especially in bacterial infections.

Eosinophile (EOS)

Appearance: Bi-lobe nucleus with red-orange cytoplasm.
Function: They are the chief cell in allergic inflammation and are also associated with parasites.

Basophile (mast cell)

Appearance: Dark granular-stained nucleus with blue cytoplasm; looks like blue pimple ball.
Function: Basophiles contain histamine, which causes vasodilatation, leading to chemosis and edema; causes hypersensitivity reaction seen in GPC, allergy, and atopic dermatitis.

Lymphocyte (lymph)

Appearance: Look like small blue balls with dark blue nucleus, with only a little cytoplasm showing.
Function: They are the chief cell in chronic inflammation.

Plasma Cell

Appearance: Eccentric nucleus; looks like a large lymph with dark blue nucleus pushed to the side; the nucleus may have a cartwheeling appearance.
Function: Plasma cells arise from B-lymphocytes. Their function is the production of antibodies.

Monocyte (macrophage or histiocyte)

Appearance: One large ovoid or horseshoe-shaped blue nucleus with dull gray-blue cytoplasm; a much larger cell than the lymphocyte.
Function: It is the major phagocytic cell in the body.

Epithelioid Cell

Appearance: Kidney-shaped nucleus with pink cytoplasm.
Function: In granulomatous disease, monocytes may be converted into epithelioid cells. They join together to form giant cells with three to six nuclei. Seen in sarcoid, trachoma, and viral infections.

(Reprinted with permission from Nemeth SC, Shea CA. *Medical Sciences for the Ophthalmic Assistant*. Thorofare, NJ: SLACK Incorporated;1988.)

17 through 22. Cell types represented in Figure 1-1: a) plasma cell, b) monocyte (macrophage/ histiocyte), c) eosinophile, d) lymphocyte, e) basophile (mast cell), f) neutrophile (PMN).

23. b) Bacteria are identified by their shape (rods, chains, etc), staining characteristics (most notably whether they are gram-positive or negative), and culture characteristics (shape, color, smell, etc). Other identifying characteristics include: size, presence or absence of a capsule, grouping or arrangement, food requirements, and oxygen requirements.

24. d) Cocci are round bacteria. They may occur alone, in pairs (diplo), in chains (strepto), or in clusters (staphylo). They may be gram-positive or negative.

25. a) The bacteria listed are all bacilli, rod-shaped bacteria. They may be gram-positive or negative, short or long, broad or thin, straight or curved. They may occur singly, in pairs, or in chains.

26. c) *Treponema pallidum*, which causes syphilis, is a gram-negative spirochete with a flagellum (whip-like tail appendage). *Staph* and *Strep* are gram-positive cocci; *H. zoster* is a virus.

27. b) Certain viruses and *Chlamydia* cause the formation of intracellular structures (usually surrounded by a clear zone) known as inclusion bodies. In the case of viruses, these usually represent viral particles. Inclusion bodies may occur in the cell's cytoplasm, nucleus, or both, and stain with Giemsa stain.

See Table 11-2 for Explanations to Questions 28 through 33.

28. d)

29. d)

30. b)

31. a)

32. b)

33. a)

See Table 11-3 for information on stains.

34. a) The envelope is a membrane that covers the cell wall. Its chemistry determines whether or not a cell will absorb or resist various stains.

35. a) These properties of a bacterium are determined by the characteristics and composition of the cell's membrane. These characteristics determine whether or not a cell will accept or resist a particular stain.

36. c) The Gram stain is the main stain used in identifying most bacteria.

37. d) A gram-negative bacterium has a cellular envelope that does not absorb the Gram stain. If the bacterium *does* absorb the Gram stain, it is gram-positive.

38. a) Gram-negative organisms appear red. Gram-positive organisms stain a dark blue.

39. d) Fungi (such as *C. albicans*) are gram-positive and will thus stain a dark blue.

40. c) The Giemsa stain is used to identify chlamydial inclusions.

41. a) Giemsa and Wright stains are used to identify the type of inflammatory cells present in a smear. Cell types are differentiated by their location and their staining properties. Certain types of cells are implicated in certain kinds of inflammatory disorders, so identification can play an important role in diagnosis.

42. d) Methylene blue is a stain for identifying fungi. Some sources also list Gram stain for this function.

43. c) India ink is sometimes used to stain the background of a slide, providing higher contrast so that the organism is more visible. The cell's capsule resists the ink so it appears clear. The cells themselves appear purple. The background is black.

44. a) *S. pneumoniae* has a polysaccharide cell capsule that resists India ink. (See Question 43.) *Candida* is a fungi.

Table 11-2
Common Bacterial Ocular Infections

Organism	Microscopic Form	Gram Stain	Culture Medium	Colonies in Culture	Pathology	Potential Findings
Staphylococcus	cocci in cluster, but may vary	+	any nutrient	opaque, round, smooth, raised, glistening, 1 to 2 mm diameter	pyogenic, necrotizing	blepharitis, hordeolum, conjunctivitis, keratitis, cellulitis
Streptococcus	cocci in chains	+	enriched (blood)	pinpoint, grayish, 2 to 4 mm zone where blood in medium has been digested	watery discharge, diffuse, spreads rapidly, often associated with injury	cellulitis
S. pneumonia (pneumonia)	lancet-shaped diplococci	+	blood agar	small, depressed in center, shiny, surrounded by zone of green	stringy discharge, invasive, edema, sudden onset	hypopyon, keratitis, chronic dacrocystitis, conjunctivitis (acute)
Neisseria gonorrhea (VD)	paired kidney-shaped intracellular organism		chocolate or blood agar	clear, glistening, large irregular edges	purulent discharge, localized	ophthalmia neonatorum, conjunctivitis, marginal corneal ulcer
Neisseria meningitidis	small, paired		chocolate or blood agar	round, low, convex, glistening, gray or gray/blue tinge	petechial or purpuric skin rash	corneal ulcer
Neisseria catarrhalis	paired		chocolate or blood agar	white, smooth, and opaque	normal throat species	conjunctivitis
Corynebacterium	slender rods in pairs or short chains	+	blood agar, Tinsdale agar	gray-black colonies with brown halo	purulent discharge	conjunctivitis
Bacillus	long rods in chains	+	blood agar	flat and irregular, 4 to 5 mm in diameter, may have undulate margin	associated with injury	endophthalmitis
Mycobacterium	typical rods	acid fast	egg, Lowenstein-Jensen	smooth/rough, pigmented or nonpigmented (depends on species), generally slow-growing	immune cell infiltrate	conjunctivitis, corneal ulcer

(continued)

Table 11-2 continued.
Common Bacterial Ocular Infections

Organism	Microscopic Form	Gram Stain	Culture Medium	Colonies in Culture	Pathology	Potential Findings
Pseudomonas	single or pair, short chains or groups	–	blood agar or fluid medium	dark greenish-gray with zone of bluish-green, sweet hay-like odor	purulent destructive necrosis	severe hypopyon, keratitis, endoph-thalmitis, corneal abcess, cellulitis
Haemophilus	tiny slender rod, no particular arrangement	–	chocolate or blood agar	pinpoint, translucent, glistening	mucoid discharge	conjunctivitis (epidemic)
Moraxella	paired	–	enriched blood	small, pinpoint (less than 0.5 mm)	subacute or chronic catarrhal	conjunctivitis, endoph-thalmitis
Treponema pallidum (syphilis)	slender, curved, flagellated	not used	no *in vitro* growth	none	3 stages	primary: chancres secondary: ulcerative blepharocon-junctivis tertiary: gummas

(Reprinted with permission from Van Boemel GB. *Special Skills and Techniques.* Thorofare, NJ: SLACK Incorporated;1999.)

45. b) Acid-fast bacteria such as *M. tuberculosis* will be a vivid red color because they retain a staining chemical used in the process that other bacteria do not.

See Table 11-4 for information on culture media.

46. c) Agar is a gel-like substance derived from red marine algae. It contains nutrients necessary for the growth of many bacterial types. Agar can be poured into petri dishes (plates) or test tubes. If test tubes are used, the tubes are slanted before the gel sets up. This slant gives more surface area on which the bacteria can grow. Broth is a liquid nutrient.

Table 11-3
Stains

Stain	Indication(s)	Notes
Giemsa	Cell stain, Chlamydial inclusions	Takes about 1 hour
Wright	inflammatory cells	Takes about 15 minutes
Gram	bacteria	Gram-negative are red, gram-positive are blue, all fungi are gram-positive
Methylene blue	Fungi	
Acid-fast	*Mycobacterium*	Acid-fast bacteria stain, a vivid red
India ink	*S. pneumoniae*	Viewed under dark illumination

Table 11-4
Culture Media

Medium	Purpose
Blood agar plate	Aerobic and facultatively anaerobic bacteria; fungi
Chocolate agar plate	Aerobic and facultatively anaerobic bacteria; enhances the isolation of *Moraxella, Neisseria, Hemophilus*
Sabouraud dextrose agar plate with Chloramphenicol or gentamicin (50 g/mL of medium)	Fungi
Supplemented Thioglycolate broth	Aerobic and anaerobic bacteria
Supplemental brain-heart infusion broth with gentamicin (50 g/mL of medium)	Fungi
Lowenstein Jensen agar slant	*Mycobacteria, Nocardia*
Thayer Martin agar plate	*Neisseria gonorrhoeae*

(Reprinted with permission from Nemeth SC, Shea CA. *Medical Sciences for the Ophthalmic Assistant.* Thorofare, NJ: SLACK Incorporated;1988.)

47. b) Certain organisms have nutritional requirements beyond what is available in plain agar. To encourage the growth of these organisms, other substances are added to the medium. These might include extracts of beef or sheep's blood, yeast, and soybean. Dextrose, sodium chloride (salt), and peptone may also be added.

48. a) Chocolate agar is blood agar heated until it is a brown color.

49. a) While *N. gonorrhoeae* may be grown on chocolate or blood agar, Thayer Martin medium is best because it enhances the growth of *N. gonorrhoeae* while retarding the growth of other bacteria that may be present.

50. d) While fungi will grow on most laboratory media, Sabouraud is preferred because it is slightly acidic (5.6) and contains lots of glucose, both of which encourage fungal growth.

51. a) The idea with any culture is to grow the causative organism and avoid contamination with other organisms. The antibiotic will discourage bacterial growth, allowing the fungus to grow alone.

52. a) Tiny-filter paper disks impregnated with antibiotic are placed on the surface of the agar plate after the plate has been streaked. If an organism is sensitive to the antibiotic in the disk, there will be a clear ring around the disk where the organism will not grow. The size of this clear ring indicates the organism's sensitivity (ie, a large ring would indicate higher sensitivity than a small ring). If no ring is present, the organism is not responsive to that antibiotic.

53. d) Any of the situations named may warrant a culture to identify the causative organism.

54. c) Viruses are very difficult to culture. They require an appropriate living host. Positive growth is established if the chick embryo dies, or by the presence of a plaque on the membrane. Tissue (or cell) cultures are cheaper and easier to use. The infected cells are evaluated to discover what effect the virus has had on them. Such effects could include ballooning (fluid accumulates in the cell), lysis (destruction of the cell), fusion of cell membranes, or malignant changes.

55. a) *M. contagiosum* is caused by a virus (see Question 54).

56. d) To obtain a conjunctival culture, do not instill anesthetic. For one thing, the procedure is only mildly uncomfortable at worst. For another, the anesthetic may be contaminated (introducing a false microbe into the study), may dilute the culture sample, or may have an antiseptic effect. Rub a moistened swab across the conjunctiva of the lower fornix, obtaining any exudate present. Avoid the lid margin. (If the lid margin needs to be cultured, it would be done separately.) Note that this procedure is different from a *scraping*.

57. a) A corneal ulcer can be sight-threatening, and may be scraped to evaluate under the microscope for microorganisms and cells. An abrasion, even from an unknown source, would not generally be cultured unless and until there was an obvious infection or ulcer.

58. a) The patient would hardly be able to tolerate a corneal scraping without topical anesthetic. The spatula is heated to sterilize it, but allowed to cool before use. Material is obtained by passing the spatula across the base or edges of the ulcer in one direction only.

59. b) Debris should be removed from the lid prior to obtaining material for a smear or culture. Use a swab moistened (but not dripping) with sterile saline.

60. d) An anterior chamber tap may be used to remove material from the chamber for culturing. Any excised tissue might be cultured. Material from any of the meibomian glands, etc, may be obtained by first cleansing the area then expressing any secretions or concretions from the structures.

61. d) All of the above procedures apply. Material obtained from the eye for cultures or smears is potentially hazardous. Universal precautions should be followed.

62. a) Growth rates can be accurate only when the date of inoculation is known. Also, the origin of the material must be noted. The same information should be noted in the patient's chart.

63. a) While labeling is mandatory, some labs inoculate plates with an L (indicating left eye) or R (for right eye) for easy identification. However, some labs use L and R only with conjunctival cultures. Other inoculating patterns include "C" for a corneal scraping and squiggly lines to indicate a lash margin culture.

64. a) The material should be spread thinly on the center of the slide before it has a chance to dry out. If it is in clumps, add a little sterile water to thin it out. On the microscope, the slide will be illuminated from behind. Viewing will be difficult if the smear is thick.

65. a) The elements of a smear are hardened and preserved quickly by fixing. This is done rapidly with the idea of preserving the tissue elements "as they were" in the body.

66. d) All three techniques are methods of fixing a smear. The method chosen depends on the type of stain to be used. Choosing the incorrect fixing method could ruin the staining procedure.

67. d) Smears meant for Gram staining are fixed by gentle flaming. Giemsa stain smears are fixed in methanol for 1 minute or dried in air. If Wright stain is to be used, the slide is allowed to air dry.

68. c) There is no such single dye known as Gram stain. The term refers to the entire process, which includes the items listed.

69. a) The cells must first be fixed (see Questions 65 and 66). Crystal violet is applied, which stains all cells. After rinsing, Gram's iodine is added to deepen the dye reaction. After another rinse, ethyl alcohol or acetone is used to decolorize the smear (see Question 71). After another rinse, safranin is used to recolor the gram-negative organisms. This is followed by a final rinse and blot-drying.

70. a) Gentian violet and Gram's iodine may be applied for 30 to 60 seconds, but the time that the smear is exposed to either should be the same.

71. d) The alcohol or acetone causes gram-positive cells to capture the violet stain (from the iodine). However, it washes out the color from gram-negative cells. If left on too long, even gram-positive bacteria will loose the dye. It is applied for only 1 to 2 seconds.

72. a) Because the ethyl alcohol or acetone decolorizes gram-negative organisms, they would be hard to see under the microscope. Safranin is a counterstain that is taken up by these microbes, enhancing their visibility with a color that is different from the dye taken up by the gram-positive organisms.

73. b) The Wright stain takes less than 15 minutes. The Giemsa stain requires 40 to 60 minutes. (Wright and Giemsa are both used to stain cell types.)

74. c) Other dilutions I discovered in research include 1 drop stain in 2 cc of water and 1.5 cc of stain in 5 cc of water.

75. a) Generally, the diluted stain is poured into a Coplin jar and the slide is immersed for 40 to 60 minutes.

76. d) The slide is next rinsed with 95% ethyl alcohol twice, for about 5 seconds each time. (Another source said tap water could be used.)

77. a) The Wright stain is left on the slide for 1 minute.

78. c) Water (most sources list distilled water) is carefully *added to* the stain on the slide in equal amounts (ie, if you used 10 drops of stain, you should dilute with 10 drops of water). The diluted solution is allowed to remain on the slide for 10 minutes.

79. a) After the diluted solution and floating residue are carefully tipped off the slide, the slide is rinsed (again, some sources say with distilled water and others say tap is okay) and allowed to air dry.

80. a) The swab is gently streaked over the agar surface. Normally the surface should not be broken or stabbed. (A *stab culture* is done for anaerobic bacteria, which are seldom seen in ocular disease.) The surface may be swabbed in a specific pattern, or it may be inoculated in a cross-hatch or squiggle pattern.

81. c) The inoculated agar plate (ie, petri dish) is placed upside down, agar side up. This is to prevent moisture from condensing the agar surface.

82. a) The rim of the tube is flamed, the swab inserted and broken off, then the rim is flamed again. A sterile swab and sterile gloves should be used. Ideally, the stick is broken off below the point where it was handled but long enough to remain above the broth. The cotton-tipped applicator is immersed in the broth.

83. a) Incubators for most bacteria are set around 35 to 37 degrees C. (Fungi are incubated at room temperature [25 degrees C].)

84. a) If there is scant growth in the first 24 hours, the physician is notified and the culture returned to the incubator. Most colonies are best evaluated during the first 48 hours, because after that they may begin to degenerate.

85. d) All of the listed features are important. Certain bacteria have unique culture qualities that help identify them. Media changes include clear zones around the colonies (where the bacteria have broken down certain medium components) or liquefaction (because the bacteria have broken down the gel).

86. a) *Aspergillus* is found in soil, water, air, and animal products. It frequently invades the lab, causing contaminating colonies to ruin bacterial cultures. It is white and feathery-looking. Older colonies are often green. Aspergillosis infection of the eye is rare, but known; blepharitis, dacryocystitis, or orbital involvement have been described.

87. d) Even in an optimal medium, fungi grow slowly. It may take 2 to 4 weeks to get fungal growth that would compare to the bacterial growth seen in only 24 hours. The same is true of viral cultures.

88. a) These cultures must be kept cold (preferably frozen) during transportation; however, dry ice is not called for.

Chapter 2. Advanced Tonometry

1. d) The indirect ischemic theory suggests that the blood flow to the nerves is reduced by pressure from the elevated IOP.

2. b) The direct mechanical theory suggests that the elevated IOP puts the squeeze on the nerve fibers themselves. (The indirect ischemic theory and the direct mechanical theory are the two most accepted ideas about how glaucoma nerve damage occurs. Most clinicians believe that damage is actually due to a combination of these effects.)

3. a) The degeneration of the trabecular meshwork as seen in glaucoma is *not* a product of the normal aging process. It seems to be disease-specific. Obstruction by particulate matter would be a secondary glaucoma. While overproduction of aqueous does exist, it is not the primary entity in open-angle glaucoma.

4. d) This was really an anatomy question. The pars plicata and ciliary processes are part of the ciliary body. These structures are damaged in chronic glaucoma.

5. c) Prolonged, elevated IOP can cause scleral thinning in the adult. This finding also occurs in children with congenital glaucoma.

6. a) Glaucoma damage to the inner retina mainly affects the nerve fiber layer and the ganglion cell layer.

7. a) The nerve fibers pass through the sieve-like lamina cribrosa. Glaucoma damage seems to be centered here. One theory regarding glaucoma damage (the mechanical theory, see Question 2) says that the lamina cribrosa is mechanically bowed by the pressure, obstructing the fibers.

8. c) Research statistics by Armaly indicated that 73% of early defects occur in the Bjerrum area. Drance's research indicated 77%. Other defects listed by the two authors as exhibiting early defects (although obviously not as frequent) were nasal steps (inside the central 30 degrees or in the periphery), concentric contraction, temporal wedges, and a combination of paracentral scotomas and nasal steps. *Other Notes*: A patient is 1.5 times more likely to have an early defect in the superior field vs the inferior field. Superior field defects may be quite developed before any defect becomes evident in the lower field. Glaucoma does not respect the vertical midline.

9. d) Once defects are present in the superior and inferior fields, the chance that the remaining visual field can be saved is poor.

10. a) The key to this answer is that the central 10 degrees has been preserved. The patient may retain 20/20 vision if there is no other ocular disease present. This phenomenon is what has earned glaucoma the title of "The Sneak Thief of Sight."

11. c) Each state has guidelines stating what extent of visual field is needed in order to drive legally. It would be more than 10 degrees in *any* state. Such a patient would qualify as legally blind on basis of restricted visual fields.

12. a) Once the patient reaches this point of visual loss, it takes only a short period of elevated IOP to rapidly eliminate (or "snuff out") the island. Thus, there is generally an attempt to keep the IOP extremely low.

13. a) Color vision and contrast sensitivity are altered in the presence of glaucoma. (The changes in color vision tend to be in the blue or blue-yellow range.) Whether or not changes in color vision and/or contrast sensitivity can be reliably used to identify glaucoma damage prior to the appearance of visual field defects is highly controversial, but it bears knowing about.

14. d) In early field loss, defects may be so shallow as to escape detection or to seem to move and appear or disappear at repeated tests. Thresholds may be unstable as well. These features make early diagnosis difficult.

15. c) Secondary glaucoma can be classified according to the location of the causative problem in relation to the trabeculum. Pre-trabecular secondary glaucoma is caused by an entity that overlies the trabeculum, such as a membrane. Trabecular secondary glaucoma involves particles (such as pigment particles, red blood cells, or inflammatory cells) or entities within the trabecular meshwork. This might occur in leukemia or sickle-cell disease, where cells might clog the meshwork. Post-trabecular secondary glaucoma occurs beyond the trabeculum, such as elevated episcleral venous pressure. The post-trabecular variety might occur in Sturge-Weber syndrome.

16. d) While medications and/or laser may be used initially to help control the IOP, the main goal in secondary glaucoma is to discover the source disorder that is causing the pressure elevation. Once the source is treated and eliminated, IOP often returns to normal.

17. a) A hypermature cataract that has "sprung a leak" is exuding liquefied cortex. Proteins from the exudate may lodge in the trabeculum. Such a cataract does not generally dislocate. Another lens-induced secondary glaucoma (unrelated to cataract) can occur in exfoliative or pseudoexfoliative syndromes, where exfoliated material from the anterior surface of the lens collects in the trabecular meshwork and obstructs aqueous outflow.

18. a) Neovascularization in the anterior chamber is most associated with diabetes. In this case, the blood vessels invade the chamber and block the angle.

19. d) Steroids do not cause a rise in IOP in every patient, but those patients who do experience an IOP increase while on steroids are known as steroid responders.

20. a) Systemic steroids can also cause elevated IOP in sensitive individuals. Drugs other than corticosteroids that may increase IOP include: anticholinergics, amphetamines, and tricyclic antidepressants.

21. a) If a pocket of aqueous has leaked into the vitreous, the volume of fluid present in the vitreous chamber is increased. This causes a flattened anterior chamber where the angle is closed off.

22. c) Pigmentary glaucoma, as the name implies, occurs when pigment is deposited in and clogs the trabecular meshwork. This pigment comes from the iris and may also be deposited elsewhere in the eye (on the corneal endothelium in the case of Krukenberg's spindles). There may be an iris transillumination defect where the pigment is missing from the iris.

23. a) Research indicates that a normal cup might withstand elevated pressures (even up to 30 mmHg) for years without field loss. Conversely, some eyes (especially if nerve damage has already occurred) experience further damage even if the IOP is in the normal range. (Once damage has occurred, it seems to take much less to cause damage. Thus, in the presence of a large c/d, some patients will experience field loss even with low IOPs.)

24. b) Ocular hypertension is generally unrelated to high blood pressure. The key in the definition of ocular hypertension is that no nerve or visual field damage has occurred at all, *not* where it has remained stable.

25. a) The patient with ocular hypertension is often labeled a "glaucoma suspect." Out of 1000 patients who carry this diagnosis, 5 to 10 will develop glaucoma each year. (This comes from Vaughan. See Bibliography.)

26. c) Malformation of the trabeculum and Schlemm's canal, in the absence of other congenital ocular abnormalities, is called isolated congenital glaucoma. Secondary (or acquired) glaucoma is due to outside causes. Secondary congenital glaucoma may be caused by trauma, inflammation, or ocular tumors. A third division exists in which the glaucoma is associated with other congenital anomalies that may be system-wide (including Down syndrome, Marfan's syndrome, Sturge Weber syndrome, and neurofibromatosis) or ocular (including aniridia and congenital cataract).

27. d) The infant with photophobia, blepharospasm, and epiphora should be seen and evaluated for glaucoma. The manifestations of isolated congenital glaucoma are usually present at birth, but may become evident during the child's first 2 years.

28. a) Elevated IOP in the infant may stretch the sclera, causing the eye to be enlarged and distended. This condition is known as buphthalmos.

29. a) The average newborn cornea is 9.8 mm in diameter (Wang). If an infant's cornea is larger than 10.5 mm, this will raise suspicions of glaucoma. (This is not to be confused with megalocornea, where the corneal diameter is greater than 13.00, but no disease state is present. Also, in megalocornea, the cornea is clear. In congenital glaucoma, there is often clouding in the central or peripheral cornea.)

30. b) The IOP of a newborn is generally under 16 mmHg (Wong, Dickens, and Hoskins). If an infant's IOP measurement is over 18 mmHg, this is suspicious of glaucoma.

31. a) Congenital glaucoma is generally treated surgically rather than with medication. One source (Vaughan) says that goniotomy is successful in producing permanent IOP control in over 85% of patients. This is true when the patient is diagnosed early. In later diagnoses, goniotomy tends to be less successful, and trabeculotomy (or trabeculectomy) is attempted.

32. b) A low-displacement tonometer does cause a slight elevation of IOP when applied to the eye, but that elevation is insignificant (eg, 5% or less). The Goldmann tonometer is a type of low-displacement tonometer. An example of a high-displacement tonometer (which displaces a large amount of aqueous, thus elevating the IOP) is the Schiotz. Low-displacement tonometers are more accurate.

33. a) The Imbert-Fick principle states that the pressure inside a sphere can be measured by applying an equal amount of pressure on the outside of the sphere.

34. a) The fixed area applanation tonometers measure the amount of force required to flatten a given area of cornea. (Fixed force tonometers measure the *amount of flattening* produced by a given force.) The area of cornea that is flattened by the Goldmann or Perkins tonometer is 3.06 mm. (The probe tip is 7 mm in diameter. The diameter of the applanated area is 3.06 mm.) During Goldmann tonometry, the force of the tears (pulling the tonometer toward the cornea and artificially lowering the measurement) and the elasticity of the cornea (resisting the tonometer and artificially elevating the measurement) cancel each other out when the proper area is flattened. When 3.06 mm of cornea is flattened, the opposite forces of the tears and cornea cancel each other out. (That's why 3.06 mm was chosen!)

35. a) The non-contact tonometer is a form of applanation tonometry. This may not be apparent at first, since there is no physical contact between the tonometer and cornea. However, the non-contact tonometer does measure the amount of force (generated by the puff) required to flatten a given area of the cornea (detected by the instrument's optics). Manometry measures the IOP directly by inserting a canula into the anterior chamber.

36. a) This minute amount of aqueous displacement (0.5 microliters) makes the Goldmann tonometer so accurate. The measured IOP is only 3% higher than the undisturbed IOP; this amount is small enough to be disregarded.

37. a) Indentation tonometry exists on the principle that the soft eye (ie, low or normal pressure) will indent more easily than a hard eye (ie, with elevated IOP). The Schiotz is the most commonly used indentation tonometer and while it might be stretching things just a bit to consider the fingers a tonometer, using the finger to judge the eye's resistance to pressure does use the principles of indentation tonometry.

38. d) For each 0.05 mm that the plunger extends beyond the footplate, the pointer moves up 1 unit on the scale. Thus, in a softer eye the plunger extends further and the gauge reads higher.

39. b) The harder the eye, the higher the eye's resistance and the lower the gauge reading on the Schiotz. While the gauge is linear, one cannot read the IOP directly from it. Also, the IOP is

not proportional to the gauge reading. Rather, the higher IOPs are clustered at the bottom of the scale. (They are clustered so tightly below a gauge reading of 3 that additional weights must be added to spread the measurements out enough to get a more exact reading.) The relationship in question is more or less logarithmic.

40. b) Theoretically, although the instrument *scale* readings would vary, when one converted the readings to an IOP measurement via the charts, the IOP would be the same with each weight.

41. c) The *weights* are specific to that instrument, not the conversion tables. The conversion tables were developed by Friedenwald using cadaver eyes. A canula attached to a reservoir was inserted into the eye so that the internal pressure of the eye could be changed at will. The tables are based on normal scleral rigidity, which is why the Schiotz is inaccurate in cases of high or low scleral rigidity.

42. b) The cornea with edema or scarring generally tends to be more elastic than normal. Thus, it takes less pressure (from the tonoprism) to applanate the required 3.06 mm. Therefore, the measurement would be lower than actuality. On a "regular" cornea, it is possible to get accurate readings without fluorescein.

43. d) The higher scleral rigidity in an eye with a scarred cornea will give a lower scale reading (because of the increased resistance) and thus an erroneously high IOP measurement.

44. d) If the cornea is irregular, the mires will also be irregular. This makes it tough to tell when the inner edges are meeting.

45. d) The Mackay-Marg tonometer is the most accurate in this case because corneal elasticity does not figure into the measurement. The Goldmann and NCT are inaccurate if the cornea has edema, scarring, or irregularities (See Question 42).

46. d) Because the Mackay-Marg and Tono-Pen measure the end point electrically (rather than optically, as with the non-contact or Goldmann/Perkins) and are not affected by corneal elasticity, the IOP can be taken through a soft contact lens. Anesthetic is used and fluorescein is not ... but these factors make no difference in this case.

47. d) This opinion comes from Brubaker in his excellent article entitled *Tonometry* (see Bibliography). Other sources agree.

48. c) The "magic number" is 3 D when it comes to resetting the tonoprism. Failure to do so may result in an erroneous measurement. (See Questions 49 and 50 for more information.)

49. b) If the biprism is not adjusted properly for the astigmatic cornea (over 3 D), the IOP measurement could be 2 to 3 mmHg off.

50. d) Turn the biprism so that the axis (in minus cylinder) is in line with the red mark on the tonometer holder. It is best to get the cylinder reading from the keratometer rather than the patient's glasses prescription, since the glasses may also correct for lenticular astigmatism. *Note*: Some sources say to turn the biprism 45 degrees from flattest the axis ... which *is* the point indicated by the red line on the holder.

Chapter 3. Advanced Visual Fields

1. d) The kinetic target is moved at a rate of 4 to 5 degrees per second (or about 0.25 inch per second). A constant, steady rate is important for accurate testing. If the target is moved too quickly, false contraction of the field can occur. It the target is moved too slowly, the isopter will be falsely large. In addition, the examination will take longer, which contributes to patient fatigue.

2. b) Because kinetic perimetry establishes a boundary by using a moving target, it is *assumed* that all areas inside the isopter will also respond to the target used to identify the isopter's border. All areas inside the isopter are also assumed to respond to any targets that are larger and/or brighter than the border-producing target. These assumptions are a weak point in the kinetic method.

3. b) Because kinetic perimetry establishes a boundary, a defect will be manifested by an irregularity in that boundary (vs normal). This could be evidenced as an inward shift of the entire boundary (constriction) or a shift of part of the boundary. Testing a single spot would be static perimetry.

4. c) The Armaly-Drance method of glaucoma screening uses both kinetic testing (to determine the boundaries of isopters) and static testing (to detect the presence of scotomas, especially in the central and nasal areas). This method is the basis for most automated glaucoma testing, but can also be used in manual perimetry.

5. d) All of the answers listed are items in the argument for static perimetry. Static perimetry (of the automated variety) is quicker, thus there is less patient fatigue and (presumably) better accuracy. Additionally, there is less patient delay in response time. (In kinetic perimetry, the patient tends to hesitate more, waiting for the target to get "close enough" to make a *definite* identification, rather than giving a first impression of seeing the target.) Defects within an isopter might well go undetected if only kinetic methods are used. In addition, thresholds within Bjerrum's area can be found. Finally, because it is more difficult to see a stationary target vs a moving one (a moving target creates the illusion of a larger target), it is considered more sensitive.

6. a) Static threshold perimetry with the Goldmann perimeter requires a static projection device as well as an intensity ruler. Threshold is determined along a single meridian. Testing is begun using a stimulus too dim to be seen; intensity is increased in 1 dB steps until it is visible to the patient. Threshold is checked every 3 to 5 degrees unless a depression is noted; in that case, every 1 to 2 degrees is checked.

7. c) In static testing of a single point, when a stimulus of a given intensity is not seen, the stimulus intensity is increased until it is seen. When the patient passes the point from not seeing the weaker stimulus to seeing the stronger, this indicates that the threshold has been crossed. The term is also used when the reverse occurs. Staircasing (or bracketing) is the *method* used to determine when the threshold is crossed, or the variation in stimulus intensity during the test such that the intensity will be suprathreshold and infrathreshold at some time during the performance of the test.

8. b) Binocular field testing is used to detect and map double vision in specific areas of gaze, a common occurrence in patients with restrictive or paralytic strabismus. It may also be used in monofixation syndrome, which involves use of red-green glasses and projectors.

9. b) Because kinetic methods are used, the Goldmann perimeter is ideal. The tangent screen can be used if the central 20 degrees of vision is not doubled.

10. c) The patient is told to *look at the target*, not at the central fixation spot. (It is important, however, that the patient only move his or her *eyes* and not the head; moving the head would alter the eyes' position and falsify the test.) Obviously, since it is a binocular test, neither eye is occluded. Corrective lenses are used if needed. The target is first shown in the central field. If the target is double, the stimulus is moved until a location is found where it is single. Single vision is mapped out in a manner similar to kinetically plotting a scotoma.

11. d) An easily seen, white stimulus is used. (This is not a test for retinal sensitivity, but rather an evaluation of extraocular muscle function.)

12. c) Diplopia that occurs outside of the central 30 degrees is generally not considered disabling (although it may disqualify one from driving, etc). An exception is if it occurs in the inferior meridians, where it can interfere with reading. Diplopia *within* the central 30 degrees is considered disabling.

13. b) The damage from toxicity is generally to the retinal layer (including the rods and cones, as well as the nerve fiber region). At the retinal level, one sees paracentral and centrocecal defects.

14. a) The papillomacular bundle is most often affected by lead poisoning, methyl alcohol, drugs (the reference, Garber's *Visual Field Examination*, did not say specifically which drugs), and digitalis. The macula can be affected by chloroquine (Plaquenil, Sanofi Winthrop Pharmaceuticals). Another reference (Glaser) listed streptomycin, chloromycetin, Antabuse (Ayerst Laboratories Inc, Philadelphia, Pa), certain drugs used to treat tuberculosis, toluene (from sniffing glue), 5-fluorouracil (5-FU, used in treating cancer), and heavy metals as toxic entities affecting the visual field, but did not say what part of the eye was affected. Glaser also listed central scotomas as a visual field defect found in these toxicities. He put forth, however, that the alcohol-tobacco amblyopia (sometimes noted under visual field defects) was more related to the poor nutritional state of the patient rather than substance use.

15. d) While noted in Question 14 that some researchers think that tobacco-alcohol amblyopia is due to poor nutrition rather than toxins, the centrocecal scotoma (which includes the blind spot and central fixation) is still considered to be associated with these conditions.

16. a) Because the papillomacular bundle or macula are the areas generally affected, vision decrease and abnormal color vision are often associated with toxicity, as well as the visual field defects.

17. a) This is easier to understand if you think of a topographic map (which is what the hill of vision is). The isopter lines (horizontal lines through the island) of a *slope* indicate a gradual falling off or a gradual decrease in sensitivity as one approaches the periphery.

18. c) If a slope is steep, the lines (horizontal slices through the island) will be closer together. If the slope is actually a drop-off, the lines will actually overlap. Conversely, in a gradual slope, the lines would be spaced farther apart.

19. a) The slope of the island of vision is steeper on the nasal side. The temporal side shows a more gradual decrease in sensitivity.

20. b) A gradually progressing lesion would likely produce a gradually sloping margin. Steep slopes are often associated with acute conditions (Pavan-Langston says these are often vascular in origin). However, reviewer Choplin notes that steep slopes may also be seen in well-established, chronic conditions which are now stable, such as strokes, or tumors which have stopped growing or have been removed.

21. d) We tend to think of an absolute scotoma as having absolutely no vision or response to a target of any intensity. However, in the strictest sense, the best you can say for sure is that the area failed to respond to the brightest stimulus available on that particular perimeter.

22. a) Once an isopter is mapped out, it is initially assumed that any point *within* that isopter will respond to the same stimulus used to map the boundary. An area within the isopter that does not respond to the initial stimulus is defined as a scotoma. If the area does *not* respond to any stimulus (even the largest and brightest) available on the instrument, it is an absolute scotoma. However, if the area *does* respond to a larger or brighter stimulus, the scotoma is referred to as relative. (See Question 29 regarding positive and negative scotomata.)

23. b) With a retinal hole, there may be loss of photoreceptors with reduced sensitivity, therefore the scotoma may be total or absolute.

24. b) A nasal step may show up first as a notch, where there is a depression at 180 degrees and the superior field is not yet contracted.

25. a) The nerve fibers of the retina arch outward from the optic nerve, but do not cross a "line" known as the horizontal raphe. Therefore, nerve fiber damage does not cross the raphe either and stops at the 180 degree mark. If fiber loss is unequal superiorly and inferiorly, a step defect occurs.

26. d) Garber's *Visual Field Examination* defines a nasal step as a 10 degree difference between the upper and lower isopters. However, if a paracentral scotoma also exists, then the definition is reduced to a 5 degree difference.

27. a) Nasal step defects are classically identified with glaucoma, although they can occur with any disc-based pathology.

28. d) Each of the listed features are important when dealing with scotomata. Density is evaluated to discover if the defect is relative or absolute (see Question 22). In addition, parts of the scotoma may have different densities. The size of the scotoma is more indicative of the degree of nerve damage. Its shape may give an indication of what type of disease process is occurring. The scotoma's position may also be related to the disorder. For example, Bjerrum scotomata are nearly always due to glaucoma.

29. a) Garber's *Visual Field Examination* lists the central scotoma as the *most* common type found in nerve damage. Pavan-Langston says that arcuate scotomata, centrocecal scotomata (which also involves the central field), and junctional scotomata may also occur. (By the way, a negative scotoma is one that the patient does not notice but is evidenced on visual field testing. In contrast, a positive scotoma is one that the patient notices.)

30. a) The key word here was "unilateral." Bilateral defects generally (although not always) occur beyond the chiasm. Bilateral central scotomata are generally due to nutritional deficiencies or toxic agents (according to Laney).

31. c) A junctional scotoma occurs in the chiasm where some of the inferonasal retinal fibers from the one eye briefly loop into the optic tract of the other eye. (These particular fibers do not actually cross over. The loop is called von Willdebrand's knee.) Thus, the defect is bilateral. Since the pituitary sits right under the chiasm, a tumor might press on the area where this looping occurs and cause a junctional scotoma.

32. Labeling: a) central scotoma, b) centrocecal scotoma, c) paracentral scotoma, d) arcuate scotoma.

33. a) Simply put, papilledema is swelling of the optic nerve head due to increased intracranial pressure. Laney lists it as the most "...common pathologic condition associated with an enlarged blind spot."

34. a) Altitudinal defects (involving the superior or inferior half of the visual field) are generally due to damage before the chiasm, which tend to respect the horizontal meridian. Post-chiasmal lesions tend to respect the vertical meridian.

35. b) A drooping lid will commonly cause a decrease in the extent of the superior field. Obviously this is an artifact if one is desirous of testing the true visual field. In some cases (notably prior to blepharoplasty) the field test may be done with the drooped lid in its natural, lowered position, followed by another test done with the lids taped up. (A *superior* retinal detachment would cause a loss in the *inferior* field.)

36. d) The optic radiations fan out through the brain tissue. The inferior fibers pass through the temporal lobe. A defect in this area results in a superior homonymous defect referred to as "pie in the sky." The superior fibers pass through the parietal lobe. A defect in this area results in an inferior defect with is generally more congruous and may be a complete or incomplete quadranopsia (known as "pie on the floor"). Although altitudinal, they also respect the vertical and are post-chiasmal (an exception to the rule, see Question 34).

Chapter 4. Advanced Color Vision

1. a) The colors that the cones specifically respond to are red, green, and blue. This sensitivity comes from the cone cell's pigment. Cones that are sensitive to red (Benson calls them "red-catching cones") contain the pigment erythrolabe. Cones that absorb green ("green-catching cones") contain chlorolabe. The blue-absorbing (or "blue-catching") cones contain cyanolabe. (To help you remember which pigment is which, it helps to know the Latin color prefixes. Here are some common terms to clue you in: erythema refers to redness, chlorophyll is found in green plants, and a person who is cyanotic appears bluish.) Color vision is not totally a matter of the cones, however; some interpretation takes place in the brain.

2. c) When we describe a color, we are actually talking about three different attributes: hue, saturation, and brightness. Hue involves which wavelength predominates. For example, if most of the photons striking the cones are in the 540 nm range, we will perceive green. Saturation is

a factor of the purity of the entering wavelengths. For example, if there is a good bit of white light mixed in with red, the red will be desaturated and the color perceived as pink. Finally, brightness refers to the luminescence of the object, or the quantity of photons emanating from it. Brightness (or lack thereof) usually affects the actual appearance of the color (there are exceptions). For example, reds and oranges appear redder at low intensities and yellower at high intensities. (Note: Some references refer to brightness as *intensity*.)

3. a) If one stares at a color (eg, a red light), the color will begin to fade (desaturate). This occurs because the cones, which are being strongly stimulated, cannot manufacture enough pigment to "keep up" with the stimulation. When the light goes off (or one looks at a white background), some messages are still en route to the brain. The red cones are fatigued, and the brain is getting a stronger message from the green/blue cones. This results in the afterimage of a complementary color.

4. b) An acquired defect (as opposed to a congenital defect) tends to gradually worsen unless the cause is treated. Because an acquired defect may affect the eyes differently, each eye should be tested separately. (Congenital defects can be tested with both eyes together.) Instead of making matching errors in a specific color range, as with a congenital defect, those with acquired defects tend to make matching errors scattered all across the color wheel. (There are, of course, exceptions.)

5. d) The anomalous trichromat has all three pigments (hence the term "trichromat"), but the level of one of them is deficient. (Anomalous is Greek for irregular.) The deficiency may be mild, moderate, or severe . . . but not absent.

6. c) The described defect is a tritanomaly. Problems with blue and yellow clue you in that the defect involves the blue color pigment, signifying this as a tritan defect. However, the next key words in the question are "some difficulty." The tritanope, who totally lacks the blue-catching pigment, would be totally unable to differentiate these colors. Tritanomaly (a form of anomalous trichromatism) is a *deficiency*, not a *lack of* the blue pigment, and would thus render the task difficult (with some wrong identifications) rather than totally impossible (with identification occurring only on pure luck). Tritan defects are rare, usually acquired, and often associated with optic nerve disease or toxicity.

7. a) First, because red is normally bright, you can rule out the protan defects. (They are deficient in or missing the red-catching pigment, so the color red will not be normally bright.) Next you must choose between the deutan defects. Deuteranomaly (deficiency) occurs in about 5% of the population. Deuteranopia (absence) occurs in about 1%. X-linked means that the gene for the defect is linked to the X (male) chromosome. (Quick genetic lesson: a male is represented by XX or xx or Xx; a female by XY or xy or Xy or xY. A dominant characteristic is denoted by an upper case letter [X or Y]. A recessive characteristic is denoted by a lower case letter [x or y]. In order for a recessive characteristic to appear/have symptoms, *it can not be* paired with a dominant. Thus the xx combination is the only possibility for a deutan defect to occur . . . linking the defect to males. A female may carry the defective gene on her x chromosome, but will not exhibit symptoms (except in, maybe, 0.5% of cases) because of the Y or y chromosome. However, she can pass the x on to her children. This explanation is grossly simplified, but will give some understanding of the concept.)

8. d) There is a 50% chance that she will have a son who is color deficient. This is because she can contribute only an x chromosome to a son, since x is the chromosome for male-ness. If her x chromosome is paired with an X chromosome from the father, the boy will not be "colorblind," because of the dominant X chromosome. If her x chromosome is paired with an x chromosome from the father, the son *will* be colorblind. The 50% figure is an average. If the father is XX, they will not have any colorblind sons; if the father is xx, then every son will be colorblind. (See Question 7, above, regarding genetics.)

9. d) This one was tricky, but Answers a through c were not technically correct. We often lump red-green defects together as if they were a single entity. They are not. While protan and deutan defects both result in confusion of red and green, it is more accurate to speak of the defect, rather than the patient's actual color vision. Thus, one should differentiate between a protan or a deutan rather than saying the patient is red-green deficient. When you take the exam, be sure to read questions carefully to determine whether they are asking about the defect itself or the patient's color vision.

10. b) The suffix "anopia" means "without vision." Thus, protanopia is "without vision of the first," since the red pigment was historically described first. Deuteranopia means absence of the green pigment and tritanopia the absence of the blue. Since there are three visual color pigments, the absence of one means there are two left... hence dichromatism ("di" = two).

11. c) According to Cassin, 2% of the population has dichromatism, the majority being protanopia and deuteranopia. Apparently, the frequency of each is very close to 1% (Van Boemel); tritanopia is very rare.

12. d) In protanopia, the red hues are black and gray. The orange-yellow-greens all look yellow. Blue-green is also grayish. Blue is more or less blue, but looks about the same as purple. The deuteranope sees red and yellow-green as the same orange-ish tone. Red-orange, orange, and yellow are all the same strong red-orange color. Magenta and green are gray tones. Blue-green to purple are various shades of blue, some of which are also confused. Finally, the tritanope sees yellow-green through purple (which includes blue) as white and gray. Reds and greens are normal.

13. b) As the term implies, a person with monochromatism has only one (mono = one) of the three visual pigments. Because the visual pigments reside in the cones, you can rule out answer c. The blue cone monochormat has *only* the blue visual pigment. This condition is so rare, it is unlikely you will ever see one.

14. b) Nystagmus, photophobia, poor visual acuity, and electroretinographic abnormalities (in spite of a normal-appearing fundus) are generally seen in rod monochromatism. They also have no color vision, identifying all colors as shades of gray. All of this occurs because there are no functioning cones in the retina.

15. c) The cone monochromat *does* have cones, but only one color pigment (instead of the normal three). These patients usually have normal visual acuity, but no hue discrimination. They do not have nystagmus or photophobia, nor are their electroretinograms abnormal (as do and are the rod monochromats).

16. d) Achromatopsia means "without color vision" ("a" = without, "chromat" = color, "opsia" = vision). It is not a statement about the color pigments present in the eye. Thus, monochromats are achromatopsic because (although a cone monochromat *does* have one of the visual pigments) they have no color discrimination at all. Achromatopsia may also occur due to damage in the cortical areas of the brain.

17. a) The most common type of anomaloscope is the Nagel. It is used to test red-green defects. There are anomaloscopes to quantify blue-yellow defects, but these are mainly found in research facilities. Notice that the question mentioned "quantify." This is an important concept. The arrangement tests tell us the type of defect, but not its severity (hence Answers c and d are incorrect). The anomaloscope is designed to tell us whether the anomaly is mild, moderate, or severe.

18. a) First, the examiner sets the color of half the circle (the upper half). Options vary from red to yellow to green. The patient is then asked to turn the yellow control knob, manipulating the color of the lower half of the circle until both halves are matched. (The patient generally is not asked to manipulate the red-green control, although this might sometimes be needed if an exact match cannot be made otherwise.)

19. b) A person with normal color vision has a very small matching range because of a high sensitivity to green and red. The wider the patient's matching range, the more severe the defect. This is the quantifying mark of the test.

20. d) The protan is red pigment deficient, and would thus add more red in order to get a "normal" effect. The deutan, being green pigment deficient, would add more green in order to match the same yellow target. Again, the larger the range, the more severe the defect. Thus a dichromat could be identified, as well as a mild to severe protanomaly or deuteranomoly . . . but it could not differentiate between the protanomaly and protanopia (hence Answer c is wrong).

21. b) The patient may need spectacle correction, but this is not as critical as it is for the arrangement tests. The test is performed on one eye at a time. The patient should not be dilated.

22. d) The white light at the base of the instrument is used before showing the patient each test circle. This "bleaches" the retina just a little, restoring the pigments to a normal level (see Question 3).

23. a) The Farnsworth-Munsell 100-hue test is an arrangement test (actually has 85 caps, not 100) that can tell the *type* of defect, as in Answer a, but not its severity.

24. d) All of the Answers are true. The test involves four boxes, for a total of 85 caps. A person with a protan defect will make arrangement errors along the axis that passes through caps 62 to 70. Deutans make errors along the axis that passes through caps 56 to 61 and tritans through caps 46 to 52. If the patient has poor color discrimination, there may be no definite pattern.

25. a) The Desaturated plates are the same as the FM D-15, except the colors are very, very pale (desaturated). It is very difficult to tell the caps from one another or from white. Because the hues are so subtle, it may pick up defects missed on the brighter FM D-15. However, it is still quantitative, not qualitative, so it does not distinguish between mild, moderate, and severe. It would be too difficult for a small child. Van Boemel's book is the only place I have ever read about this test.

26. a) The Sloan achromatopsia test uses six very highly concentrated colors from the color wheel. The patient attempts to match these with a set of gray samples of graded shades. A person with achromatopsia can match them; a person with any color vision at all cannot. The only reference in which I found this test was Adams.

Chapter 5. Advanced Clinical Optics

1. b) The stenopaic slit is especially useful for patients with irregular astigmatism, such as those with keratoconus. The slit allows evaluation of vision along a single meridian, since it blocks out light from all other meridians (but the one). It may also be useful in patients with high astigmatism . . . or any case where the retinoscopy reflexes are confusing or poor.

2. c) A spherical lens is selected that will give a working vision. There is no cylinder present at this point.

3. a) As long as the cornea is the cause of most of the astigmatism (vs lenticular astigmatism), the first slit position where the letters are clearest corresponds to the axis of the minus cylinder. Another way to think of this is the axis of the flattest keratometric value. (*Note*: If the patient rotates the slit 180 degrees and no difference is reported, try fogging the patient by adding a little plus. This will move the circle of least confusion off of the retina. Another possibility is that the slit is not directly over the pupillary axis; reposition the trial frames.)

4. a) Put your information on a power cross. The 135 meridian has a power of 3.75. The 45 meridian has a power of 9.25. To determine the measurement, start with your first reading, which also contains the minus cylinder axis. At this point you have: 3.75 ? 135. To get the amount of the cylinder, calculate the difference between 3.75 and 9.25. The result is 5.50. Your answer: 3.75 5.50 135.

5. d) Guyton states that the three limitations, especially of early instruments, were accommodation, irregular astigmatism, and alignment. We tend to accommodate automatically when looking into any instrument; Guyton says this tendency is "known variously as instrument myopia, instrument accommodation, and apparatus accommodation."

6. a) Nearly all automated refractors use the optometer principle, which was first described by Porterfield in 1759. Guyton describes it this way: "The optometer principle . . . permits continuous variation of power in refracting instruments. Instead of interchangeable trial lenses, a single converging lens is used, placed at its focal length from the eye or . . . from the spectacle plane. Light from a target on the far side of the lens enters the eye with vergence of different amounts (zero, minus, or plus), depending on the position of the target. If the vergence of the light in the focal plane of the optometer lens is measured, it will be discovered to be linearly related to the displacement of the target." Hunter and West explain that "an illuminated mobile target is moved back and forth along the optical axis of an unknown lens . . . until the vergence leaving the lens is zero." (From this, you can see that the lensometer is also based on the optometer principle.)

7. a) The part of the retina that senses infrared light is different than the photoreceptor layer that senses visible light. Since the refractometric measurement is intended to focus visible light, the computer program of the instrument includes a conversion factor to go from invisible infrared to visible light. (Without this conversion, the measurement could be 0.75 to 1.50 D off, says Guyton.)

8. a) In subjective automated refractometry, patient responses are required. These may be oral responses to an operator (who controls the phoropter via remote control) or electronic responses to the computer that controls the phoropter (via a flow-chart type of program). Objective automated refractometry involves no response from the patient; this is what we usually think of when we hear the term "automated refractometers."

9. d) Combining the methods of objective and subjective refractometry is ideal, and most patients will be able to cooperate for the subjective portion . . . for example, first performing retinoscopy (which is objective) and then refining your reading with subjective methods ("which is better, one or two?").

10. b) Remember, subjective means that the patient's response is required. (I remember this by thinking that in objective testing, I treat the patient like an object . . . no human response is required.) Because anterior segment disease invariably involves the media, reflexes (from retinoscopy or automated refractometry) can be difficult or impossible to interpret. Subjective methods would be best in such a case.

11. Labeling:
    a) Less likely to prescribe "uncomfortable" glasses (subjective)
    b) Revelation of latent hyperopia (objective)
    b) Reveals information about the media (objective)
    b) Eliminates problems created by patient misunderstanding (objective)

12. b) If the chart is moved to 5 feet, accommodation becomes a factor. It takes +0.66 D to accommodate at 5 feet, and this amount can be subtracted after the measurement is complete. (This comes from Garber's article *Low Vision*, which says you need move the chart to 5 feet only if the patient's vision is worse than 10/200.)

13. a) Nystagmus can worsen if one eye is occluded, thus reducing the patient's potential visual acuity. Instead of covering the non-tested eye, fog it with a +6.00 lens. Because nystagmus may also be quieter in a specific gaze, use trial frames and allow the patient to position his or her head in the "quiet" field (which varies from patient to patient). It is pretty hard to do that with a phoropter.

14. a) Because low vision patients frequently need lenses of high power, thus making vertex distance a very important issue, the trial frame is the instrument of choice. In addition, objective methods do not work well in low vision patients with media problems. The trial frame also makes it easier to offer the patient larger increments when changing lenses. Low vision patients may not appreciate a 0.50 D change and require higher increments to appreciate the difference. (By the same token, a 0.50 D cross cylinder may not provide enough contrast, either. Use one that provides at least 1.00 D.) Also, if the patient has a central scotoma, the small apertures in the phoropter do not provide enough field of vision. (By the same token, full aperture trial lenses are best as well.) Finally, the trial frame allows the patient to adopt any advantageous head posture if eccentric viewing is used.

15. b) You should move the reading matter with each lens change so that it is in the focal distance for that lens. (By the way, "task-oriented reading material" means a reading card with full text, music, or number tables on it, not isolated optotypes.)

16. c) The plano soft contact lens will provide a smooth surface. This especially makes any objective measurements easier. Other options that might help are keratometry, corneal topography, and the stenopaic slit (see Question 1).

17. c) Before we embark on solving these problems dealing with simple lens systems, we need to review just a bit. The formula we need for these problems is $1/U + 1/f = 1/V$ where U is the distance from the object to the lens (in meters), f is the focal length of the lens, and V is the distance from the lens to the image (in meters). Also, light emanating from an object in front of a lens is always divergent, and therefore negative.

    First, plug into the formula. $1/ 0.50$ m $+ 1/ 0.33 = 1/V$. (Confused? Well, 50 cm must be converted to meters for the formula to work, so you get 0.50 m. Then, the focal length of a 3.00 lens is 0.33; remember diopters $= 1/$focal length.) Now dust off your algebra hat. $1/ 0.50$ equals 2; $1/ .33$ equals 3.03; so we now have $2 + 3.03 = 5.03 = 1/V$. To get the V to stand alone, first multiply both sides by V/1 (remember, you can do anything to one side of the equation as long as you also do it to the other side): $5.03 \quad V/1 = 1/V \quad V/1$. This gives you $5.03V = 1$. Next, divide both sides by 5.03: $5.03V/ 5.03 = 1/ 5.03$. This divides out so you have V $= 0.1988$. Round this up to 0.20 m. Your answers are in centimeters, though, so you have got to convert, leaving you with 20.0 cm. The minus tells you that the distance we have found is still in front of the lens. (Remember attributes of minus lenses to remember that a minus lens creates a virtual image on the same side of the lens as the object.) The next problems will not go into as much detail about solving the problem; here I just wanted to refresh your algebra!

18. b) First, plug the numbers into the formula: $1/U + 1/f = 1/V$. $1/ 2 + 1/0.15 = 1/V$. $0.50 + 6.67 = 1/V$. $+6.17 = 1/V$. V $= +0.16$ m. (The plus sign tells us that the image is on the opposite side of the lens from the object.)

19. b) Plug into the formula $1/U + 1/f = 1/V$. $1/ 3 + 1/f = 1/0.25$. $0.33 + 1/f = 4$. Subtract 0.33 from each side (same as adding $+0.33$): $1/f = 4.33$. $f = 0.23$. But you are not done yet; this is the lens' focal length, not its power. Now plug into the formula to find the power: D $= 1/0.23$. D $= +4.35$. (We also know that this is a plus lens because the image is on the opposite side of the lens from the object.)

20. c) Plug into the formula $1/U + 1/f = 1/V$. $1/U + 1/ 0.36 = 1/ 0.12$. $1/U + (2.78) = 8.33$. $1/U = 5.55$. U $= 0.18$ m.

21. d) On to compound (or multiple) lens systems. The good news is really good: we can use the same $1/U + 1/f = 1/V$ formula from above to solve multiple lens system questions. You simply treat each lens as a single lens system. (The image from the first lens simply becomes the object for the second; however, you must pay careful attention to its position to determine if it has negative or positive vergence.)

    We begin with the $+4.00$ lens, since we have been told that light enters it first. Plug into the formula: $1/ 0.5 + 1/0.25 = 1/V$. $2 + 4 = 1/V$. $+2 = 1/V$. V $= 0.5$ m.

    Thus, the $+4.00$ lens creates an image 0.5 m (or 50 cm) from itself. We now turn our attention to the second lens. However, remember the 25 cm between the first and second lenses. Thus, the *image* from the $+4.00$ lens is actually 25 cm *beyond* the $+1.00$ lens (50 cm 25 cm). This time, remember to use positive vergence instead of negative.

    Now plug into the formula again: $1/0.25 + 1/1 = 1/V$. $4 + 1 = 1/V$. $5 = 1/V$. V $= 0.20$ m.

22. b) First plug the +2.00 lens into the formula: $1/\ 4.0 + 1/0.50 = 1/V$. $0.25 + 2 = 1/V$. $1.75 = 1/V$; $V = 0.57$ m behind the +2.00 lens. But remember, the two lenses are 0.37 m apart. Thus, the image from the first lens is 0.20 m behind the second lens; this gives it positive vergence.

    Now plug in the second lens: $1/0.20 + 1/\ 0.125 = 1/V$. $5.00 + (\ 8.00) = 1/V$. $3.00 = 1/V$. $V = \ 0.33$ m. The negative indicates that the image is 0.33 m in front of the second ($\ 8.00$) lens.

23. d) Since a plane mirror is flat, it has no vergence and thus no power.

24. a) The image created by a flat mirror is virtual, erect, and not inverted from side to side. This side-to-side issue can be confusing. The image is on the opposite side of the mirror from the object, but left and right are not inverted. Imagine this: You are standing in front of a plane mirror, and a friend is behind you at your right shoulder. In the mirror, the image of your friend is to the left of your image. However, if your friend lifted his right hand, his right hand would still be on the right in the mirror. So while the image of your friend is opposite his actual location, the image is not inverted left to right.

25. c) Parrish writes, "The image of a point in front of a [plane] mirror is located behind the mirror at the same distance that the object point is situated in front of the mirror." Thus the answer is 2.0 m: 1.0 from the object (yourself) to the mirror and the apparent 1.0 from the mirror surface "back" to the image. We use this principle frequently in eyecare when we use mirrors to "extend" the length of an exam room.

26. d) The law of reflection applies to all mirrors, plane and curved.

27. b) This was not difficult if you recognized that a mirror with a virtual image on the opposite side from the object is a convex mirror. Convex mirrors have negative vergence (or "negative power"). A concave mirror has a magnified, real image on the same side of the object, as well as positive vergence (or "positive power").

28. d) A shaving mirror is concave, and thus it has a real image. Real images are inverted; however, if you are at or closer than the mirror's focal distance, the image becomes virtual and thus erect. (That is why you have to get so close to the shaving mirror.) The same thing happens with a high plus (magnifying) lens.

29. a) Start with the formula: $P = 2/(r)$, where P is the power in diopters and r is the radius of curvature of the mirror in meters. First, you must convert 100 mm to meters: 0.1 m. Now, plug into the formula: $P = 2/0.1$. The answer is +20 D. (Be sure to always look and see what type of mirror the question gives you. If this had been a convex mirror, the answer would have been $\ 20$ D because a convex mirror has negative power. [See Questions 27 and 30.])

30. b) The formula for finding focal length of any curved mirror is $F = (r)/2$, where F is the focal length in meters and r is the radius of curvature of the mirror in meters. But this question does not give you the radius of curvature, so you have to use the formula in Question 29 to find it: $P = 2/(r)$. Thus, $\ 50 = 2/(r)$, and $r = \ 0.04$ m. Now we can use the first formula. Plugging in the values, we have: $F = \ 0.04/2 = \ 0.2$ m. (Note: Instead of saying that the focal length is negative, some writers would instead note that the image is in front of the mirror.)

31. c) A convex mirror minifies objects, thus allowing for a wide field of vision . . . useful in store monitoring and driving. However, because images are minified, they appear to be farther away than they actually are. Misjudging distance could be hazardous for drivers, hence the warning.

32. d) The accommodative amplitude is the maximum amount that the lens can accommodate and is measured in diopters.

33. b) Depth of focus is often used when speaking of photography and cameras. To use the camera analogy, the camera has a lens of a fixed power. You select a single, unmoving object of interest to photograph, let's say a cat. (A sleeping cat.) The only variable is how close you stand to the cat when looking through the camera. If you get too far away, the image will be blurred. If you get too close, the image will also be blurred. The area in between the points where the image begins to blur (be it close or distant) is the lens's depth of focus. The same applies to the eye, but in this case we are strictly referring to a near object (ie, one that stimulates any accommodation that the eye may have). Thus, the range of accommodation is the distance between the far point (farthest away that the near target can be and still be seen clearly) and the near point (closest that the near target can be and still be seen clearly).

34. b) The patient's range of accommodation is the distance between the near point and far point (33 − 8 = 25). Furthermore, it is the 25 cm that fall between 8 cm and 33 cm.

35. d) First, you must convert the "points" to diopters. $F = 1/f$ where F is the far point in diopters and f is the far point in meters. $N = 1/n$ where N is the near point in diopters and n is the near point in meters. So we have $F = 1/0.33$ and $N = 1/.08$. Thus $F = 3.03$ D and $N = 12.5$ D. The amplitude in diopters equals the difference between the dioptric power of the far point and the dioptric power of the near point (12.5 − 3.03), in this case 9.47 D . . . rounded off to 9.5 D.

36. a) When measuring the patient's amplitude of accommodation, it is expected that the patient is best corrected for distance, creating emmetropia. In this situation, accommodation is relaxed up to the far point (which is infinity in emmetropia). At the near point, all available accommodation has been expended.

37. a) The +3.00 add will bring her near point onto the Prince rule. Measure her amplitude, read the dioptric value from the rule, and subtract the +3.00 lens from the results.

38. d) Any of the mentioned situations can cause the amplitudes to be unequal. You might think that anisometropia would also be a possible answer; however, a 40-year-old eye still has about 4 D of accommodative power whether it is a −2.50 or a +3.25 . . . in either eye. Any trauma severe enough to damage the ciliary muscle (eg, a penetrating injury) or rupture the zonules could also cause an accommodation problem in the affected eye.

39. b) By age 40, the lens has become stiff enough to reduce its accommodative ability to about 4 D. This means that the eye's near point is 25 cm, which is farther back than the patient is generally comfortable with. Reviewer Lens reminds us that even though the patient has 4 D of accommodative amplitude, 50% of this amplitude should be held in reserve for "comfortable" reading.

40. c) Binocular balancing is done to make sure that the accommodation of the eyes is relaxed equally. For example, if the distant refraction leaves the patient's accommodation relaxed in one eye but exerting +0.75 in the other, then the refraction is not balanced and the add will be off—properly correcting one eye but not the other. This is uncomfortable for the patient.

41. b) Actually, her range of focus with the +2.25 will be *decreased*.

42. a) In patients who have some accommodative ability left, it is generally desirous to let them use half of their natural reserve for near work and supply the other half with an add. For example, it takes about +3.00 to focus at 14 inches (rounded off). The 40-year-old patient has about 4 D of accommodative ability. Let him use half of what he has got (ie, +2.00), and provide him with an external +1.00 in the form of reading glasses. The 60-year-old with 1 D of accommodative ability should use +0.50 of her own and be given a +2.50 reading add. Obviously, this is mathematics and optics, which does not always work in the real world. But it is still a good guideline.

43. d) This is tricky, and your exam will not ask tricky questions. This is another one of those "learning experience" questions. First of all, the "X" system tells you how many times the image will be enlarged; thus, a 2X lens doubles the image, and a 6X lens multiplies it by six. The deciding factor in determining this lens's effective power was the distance at which the lens is to be used (which was not supplied in the question). In low vision, 40 cm is considered standard. In that case, the Answer would be b, or +15.00 D. However, some manufacturers use a 25 cm standard reference distance. In that case, the Answer would be c, or +24.00. (It might help you to remember that with a 25 cm reference distance, you need only multiply the X power by four to get the effective dioptric power.)

    Author's Note: This same topic is listed for the ophthalmic technician candidate under the Clinical Optics heading. You may wish to review Questions 166 through 178 in Chapter 2 of *Certified Ophthalmic Technician Exam Review Manual*. I have tried to offer you more advanced questions here, and have covered *only* optical aids.

44. c) The first number is the dioptric power (10) and the second number is the amount of base in prism (12). Beyond about 4 to 6 D, base in prism is automatically incorporated into high-powered reading glasses in order to offset the higher convergence that would be required when using high plus lenses at a close working distance. These lenses run from 6 to 12 D. Above 12 D, such lenses are referred to as microscopes instead.

45. a) The light rays emerging from the magnifier are parallel, so changing the distance between the eye and magnifier do not affect the image size or the focus. To adjust focus, one would need to change the distance between the magnifier and the reading material (object). (Magnifiers are best focused at the focal length of the lens.) One may increase the field of view by maintaining the lens-to-object distance and pulling *both* the lens and object closer to the eye.

46. a) The first number tells you how many times objects will appear to be enlarged through the telescope. The second number gives the diameter of the objective lens in millimeters. The last number tells how many degrees in the field of view, provided that the pupil is normal in size.

47. b) Telescopes provide images that appear closer than they actually are by means of angular magnification. Because of experience, the person knows that the object is not actually larger; instead, the brain interprets the image as being closer. Relative size magnification refers to literally enlarged objects, such as large print. Relative distance magnification refers to bringing objects closer in order to enlarge them. Projection magnification enlarges images, as in closed circuit TV or overhead projectors.

48. c) The makeshift telescope is created by combining a high *minus* contact lens with a high *plus* reading glass for one eye. It is used for distance viewing, but ignored when reading or moving. The remaining statements are true. The situation in Answer d works because reversing the telescope *minifies* the patient's view, providing a broader field of vision.

49. b) Prentice's rule is the formula for prism decentration.
Author's Note: "Prism correction" is listed as a content area for the ophthalmic technician candidate under the heading of Clinical Optics. You may wish to review Questions 139 through 151 in Chapter 2 of *Certified Ophthalmic Technician Exam Review Manual*.

50. c) First, you must plug the known values into the formula: Induced prism = lens power (in diopters) × optical center displacement (in centimeters); 2 prism diopters = +6.00 × OCD. This is converted algebraically to OCD = 2 prism diopters/+6.00 = 0.33 cm = 3.3 mm. In order to create base out in a plus lens, the center must be moved out.

51. a) Plus lenses that are decentered in will induce base in prism. Next figure the induced prism in each lens. OD: 2.75 D × 0.275 cm = 0.75 prism diopters. OS: 2.00 D × 0.125 cm = 0.25 prism diopters. Since both prism bases are in the same direction, their power is additive: 0.75 prism diopters + 0.25 prism diopters = 1.00 prism diopters.

52. b) Start by putting the lenses on optical crosses. Once this is done, you can see that for the right lens, you are dealing with −5.00 in the vertical, and for the left lens −4.50 in the vertical. Decentration is the same for both lenses: 3.0 mm, or 0.3 cm. Now plug into the formula. OD: 5.00 D × 0.3 cm = 1.5 prism diopters. OS: 4.50 D × 0.3 cm = 1.35 prism diopters. Vertical prism is additive only when the bases are opposite, but in this case they are the same, so you subtract: 1.5 prism diopters − 1.35 prism diopters = 0.15 prism diopters base up.

53. a) The two divisions are industrial wear and street wear. The qualification for industrial wear is given in the question. To qualify for street wear, the lens must withstand the impact of a 5/8 inch steel ball (dropped from the same height). *Note*: Plastic lenses are exempt from this test because they are already impact resistant.
Author's Note: This topic is also covered under the criteria for Certified Ophthalmic Assistant, which made it difficult to judge what material to include here.

54. c) Standards also call for an industrial safety lens to be at least 3 mm thick at the edges if a plus lens or 3 mm thick in the middle if a minus lens. For street wear safety lenses, the minimum thickness is 2.2 mm.

55. b) Polycarbonate is the preferred material for safety lenses. It is more impact resistant than any other material (even treated types). Because it has a high refractive index, polycarb lenses are also thinner and more lightweight.

56. c) The most popular schematic eye was developed by Gullstrand in the early 1900s.

57. b) The idea behind the schematic eye was to provide optical constants in order to explain the physiologic optics involved in the human ocular optical system.

58. d) See Table 11-5 for the types of information provided by Gullstrand's schematic eye.

Table 11-5
The Schematic Eye

Structure	Notes
Cornea	IR = 1.376 Radius of central anterior surface = 7.7 mm Radius of posterior surface = 6.8 mm Refractive power of anterior surface = +48.83 D Refractive power of posterior surface = 5.88 D Total refractive power = +42.95 D Central thickness = 0.5 mm
Pupil	"Ideal" size = 2 to 5 mm
Aqueous	IR = 1.336
Lens	IR of cortex = 1.386 IR of nucleus = 1.406 Overall IR = 1.42 Anterior radius of curvature (unaccommodated) = 10.00 mm Anterior radius of curvature (fully accommodated) = 5.33 mm Posterior radius of curvature (unaccommodated) = 6.0 mm Posterior radius of curvature (fully accommodated) = 5.33 mm Refractive power (unaccommodated) = +19.11 D Refractive power (fully accommodated) = +33.06 D Thickness of nucleus = 2.419 mm Overall thickness = 3.6 mm
Vitreous	IR = 1.336
Axial length	Overall eye length = 24.4 mm Distance from anterior K to anterior lens surface = 3.6 mm Distance from anterior K to posterior lens surface = 7.2 mm Distance from posterior lens surface to retina = 17.2 mm

59. b) When spheres and lenses are combined, there are two focal lines. These lines are perpendicular to each other and one is in front of the other. The space between the two lines is known as Sturm's interval (Figure 11-2).

60. d) As shown in Figure 11-2, the light rays within Sturm's interval are focused in a cone shape. This is called the Conoid of Sturm, or Sturm's conoid.

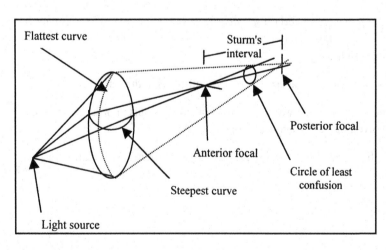

Figure 11-2. Conoid of Sturm. (Reprinted with permission from Lens A. *Optics, Retinoscopy, and Refractometry.* Thorofare, NJ: SLACK Incorporated; 1999.)

61. a) As shown in Figure 11-2, the circle of least confusion is in the center of Sturm's conoid. In front of and behind this circle, cross-sections through the conoid are ellipse shaped. While the image is not in focus at any point in the conoid, it is *most* focused at the circle of least confusion. The goal in refractometry of the astigmatic eye is to use a spherocylindrical lens to collapse Sturm's interval so that both focus lines fall on the retina simultaneously.

Chapter 6. Advanced Ocular Motility

1. b) If the eye looks normal yet has decreased vision despite treatment at an early age, the amblyopia is classified as organic. Using the term functional amblyopia implies that the poor vision is treatable.

2. c) Refractive amblyopia is generally bilateral and due to high, uncorrected refractive errors. (Reverse amblyopia is another name for occlusion amblyopia, see Question 6. Reflex amblyopia is caused by an injury or other insult to the eye. Anisometropic amblyopia develops when there is a refractive difference between the eyes.)

3. b) The child in this scenario has "natural" monovision. In such a case, even if the child is anisometropic, amblyopia might not develop. The child often uses the myopic eye for near and the hyperopic eye for distance. However, because the eyes do not see a clear image at the same time, the patient does not have perfect fusion (maybe in the neighborhood of 400 seconds). Because of the desirability of promoting fusion in childhood, the refractive correction will generally be given in some form.

4. d) Amblyopia ex anopsia is another name for amblyopia of disuse. It is also called stimulus deprivation. This is the type of amblyopia that remains once the organic cause of the poor visual development has been removed (such as congenital ptosis, congenital cataract, or anything that obscures the visual axis for a sufficient period of time). The other answers are actually types of amblyopia; see Hoffman's book or some other reference for the definitions.

5. b) In non-alternating strabismus, only one eye is being used. The other eye does not have a chance to develop visually, thereby causing amblyopia. However, when you test a child and find non-alternating strabismus, this is also a *sign* that the you can expect the non-preferred eye to be amblyopic.

6. b) If the "good" eye is patched too long, its visual development may become impaired. This results in reverse amblyopia (in other words, the amblyopia has reversed from the original eye to the "good" eye). Another term for this is occlusion amblyopia.

7. d) Cycloplegia of a mildly myopic eye will not penalize the vision in the better eye enough to force the child to use the weaker eye. (This comes from Hansen.)

8. a) The patch is best applied to the face, because the child will usually look around the glasses. Hansen says that a good rule of thumb regarding follow-up with patching is to allow 1 week for each year of the child's age (ie, a 1-year-old is rechecked in 1 week, a 2-year-old in 2 weeks, etc). Also to be considered are psychological factors (the stigma of "the patch," the responses of other children and family members, etc).

9. c) The 0.4 foil (or filter) is a denser filter. (In contrast, a 0.8 is less opaque.) It is best used when the eyes have been treated to the point where there is only a few line's difference between

the eyes yet the amblyopia persists. Hansen says that if the vision is worse than 20/50 in the amblyopic eye, foils are not advisable because the child will look around the glasses. She further states that the best candidates for foil use are older children who understand their treatment, have straight (or very nearly straight) eyes, and who are highly motivated *not* to wear a conventional patch. Using a non-opaque occlusion is also called graded or incomplete occlusion.

10. b) Hansen says that the full amount of pushed plus should be prescribed for the amblyope with an esodeviation. The amount of plus might be reduced a bit for exodeviations or orthophoria.

11. b) In *Treatment of Amblyopia*, Greenwald and Parks warn that even though initial treatment is successful, the result will not necessarily be maintained. They recommend keeping an eye on things at least until the age of visual maturity (around 10 years of age).

12. a) By optimizing the vision in the amblyopic eye prior to alignment surgery, the physician increases the chances that the eyes will be able to fuse and "lock" together, holding the eyes straight (*Treatment of Amblyopia* by Greenwald and Parks). (*Note*: Reviewer McClatchey reports that Guyton et al recently published a study showing that this is not necessary. However, he notes that most pediatric ophthalmologists still treat amblyopia first.)

13. c) In high astigmatism, it is possible for visual development to take place in the more emmetropic meridian and less development (ie, amblyopia) to develop in the most ametropic meridian. Greenwald and Parks describe this in *Amblyopia*, but also note that its effect on visual acuity is not marked. (*Notes*: Color amblyopia is another term for color vision deficiency. Suppression amblyopia is another term for stimulus deprivation amblyopia. Isoametropia is a symmetric, high refractive error, sometimes resulting in an amblyopia that may or may not be bilateral.)

14. a) The inferior oblique originates at the posterior lacrimal crest at the orbital rim margin (infero-nasally). The other five EOMs originate in the annulus of Zinn.

15. c) The spiral of Tillaux is created by the spiraling effect of the rectus muscles as they insert onto the globe. Starting with the SR and moving laterally (ie, SR, LR, IR, to MR), the distance from the limbus to the muscle insertion is 7.7 mm, 7.0 mm, 6.5 mm, and 5.5 mm, spiraling closer to the corneal as you go around. (*Note*: Different references will give slightly different measurements for the limbus to insertion distances; the spiral remains the same, regardless. My data comes from Hansen.)

16. b) The superior oblique runs through the trochlea prior to inserting on the globe. If this question seemed tricky, do not worry. The real exam is not tricky.

17. c) When the eye is in primary position, the LR and MR coincide with the eye's visual axis. Another way of saying this is to refer to their muscle plane angles as 0 degrees. The muscle plane angles of the other EOMs are as follows: SR and IR, 23 degrees; SO, 54 degrees; IO, 51 degrees.

18. a) All of the rectus muscles insert in front of the equator (see Question 15). Both obliques insert behind the equator. The SO inserts underneath the SR, and the IO inserts under the LR.

19. d) The LR is innervated by the abducens nerve (CNVI). (Remember this: the LR ABducts, and its nerve is the ABducens. Also, remember the mnemonic LR6SO4: the LR is supplied by CNVI, and the SO by CNIV. The rest are CNIII [oculomotor nerve].)

20. a) The SR is supplied by the superior division of CNIII (the oculomotor nerve). This makes sense: the *superior* rectus is supplied by the *superior* division; the *inferior* muscles are supplied by the *inferior* division.

21. a) Herring's law says that equal innervation is applied to the yoke muscles of each eye.

22. b) Sherrington's law applies to ductions. It states that the amount of innervation supplied to the agonist muscle is balanced by an equal amount of relaxation to the antagonist muscle.

23. a) Herring's law applies to binocular eye movements (versions).

24. a) Herring's law applies to binocular eye movements. In this case, the RLR is underactive. When the patient fixes with OS, OD pulls in because of the underaction of the RLR. However, it requires "extra" innervation for the patient to fix with OD. Since Herring's law tells us that equal innervation will go to the LMR, and "extra" is going to the RLR, the LMR also receives "extra." This causes the LMR to receive excessive stimulation, pulling it to overshoot (making the secondary deviation greater than the primary deviation).

25. d) Accommodation and convergence are linked. Accommodative convergence is the amount of convergence that is triggered by a specific amount of accommodation. Accommodative demand is aimed at maintaining a clear image at near; convergence demand is aimed at avoiding diplopia.

26. a) The AC/A ratio is a comparison of the amount of accommodative convergence (measured in prism diopters) generated by each diopter of accommodation.

27. b) Age definitely affects accommodation (ie, presbyopia); there is also, however, a corresponding decrease in accommodative convergence, hence a person's AC/A ratio tends to remain the same throughout life. (This according to D'Agonstino.) Of course there are always exceptions. Reviewer McClatchey notes that "children with high AC/A ET sometimes outgrow the need for bifocals, even without surgical intervention." But *most* people's AC/A is stable throughout life.

28. c) If the ratio is 8/1 (8 prism diopters of convergence per each 1 D of accommodation) and 3 D of accommodation are required, 24 prism diopters of convergence are created (3 × 8). If the normal person expends 18 prism diopters and our patient expends 24, the difference between normal and our patient is 6 prism diopters (24 − 18).

29. d) The uncorrected hyperope has to accommodate even to see at a *distance*. This accommodation stimulates convergence, since convergence and accommodation are linked together. In this case, convergence causes diplopia which the patient must struggle to overcome.

30. a) This is a standard method of measuring AC/A. In this case, A = 3 (the +3.00 lens). AC is the difference between the "with" and "without" measurements of the deviation (53 − 14 = 21). The answer is 21/3, which reduces to 7/1.

31. d) The normal angle kappa is about 2 to 4 degrees (per Vaughan, Asbury, and Riordan-Eva; Lennarson, as well as Pavan-Langston, say up to 5 degrees), because the visual axis (the point of the corneal reflection) is about 2 to 4 degrees nasal of the pupillary center. If the visual axis and pupillary center coincide (as in this example), then there is an angle kappa of zero.

32. a) A negative angle kappa means that the reflex is temporal to the pupillary center. This gives the false impression that the eye is turned in. Actually, this is an uncommon finding.

33. b) Because a positive angle kappa has a reflex that is nasal to the pupillary center, it looks like an exotropia. If the eye actually has an ET and a positive angle kappa, the ET may be masked or underestimated. Pavan-Langston says this occurs commonly in children with arrested RLF. Reviewer McClatchey adds that this usually happens in severe cases.

34. c) A perimeter may be used to measure the angle kappa; the patient fixates on the central mark and the operator moves a light until its reflex is in the center of the pupil. The degrees of difference between the center mark and the light reflex is the angle kappa. A synoptophore slide may also be used: the patient is asked to look at a specific number or figure on the slide until the reflex is centered. (Each optotype is 2 degrees apart; thus, if the light was centered when the patient looked at the fourth figure, the angle kappa would be 8. Positive or negative would depend on which side of center that the patient was looking.)

35. c) Fusional amplitude refers to the amount of prism that the patient can overcome to maintain single vision (ie, avoid diplopia).

36. b) Normal convergence amplitudes at near are 20 prism diopters (break point) and 18 prism diopters (recovery point). This is about double the distance convergence amplitudes and the near divergence amplitudes. It is over three times the distance divergence amplitudes.

37. a) When enough prism has been added to finally cause fusion to break down (resulting in diplopia), this is recorded as the break point. Once the break point has been reached, the recovery point is that prism where the patient can first re-fuse.

38. c) Stereopsis is *not* a given, even when the patient has normal binocular vision and fusion. There is a motor component to fusion; that is, the eyes' movements are coordinated in order to produce fusion. No such component exists to give us stereopsis; it is merely a benefit of fusion.

39. b) Stereoacuity should be performed first, before fusion has been broken by any other test, because it is the most sensitive fusion test. Worth four dot is next, followed by cover-uncover testing. (Hansen reminds us that the single cover-uncover test is a test for motor fusion control, not for alignment.) The visual acuity test definitely breaks fusion, and must be done *after* all fusion tests have been performed.

40. c) Central stereopsis is the stereopsis present at the fovea, where there is a point-to-point correspondence of retinal points. From fixation to 20 degrees from fixation, this is more of an area-to-area correspondence, and points that are farther apart (than central stereopsis would allow) are still fusible. Beyond 20 degrees stereopsis is poor or non-existent.

41. c) Arc disparity changes with testing distance. If held at 7.5 inches, the 40 second test object becomes 80 seconds. If held at 30 inches, it becomes 20 seconds.

42. c) In evaluating nystagmus, the speed of each movement, its amplitude, and its duration in each direction are considered. Pendular nystagmus could be compared to the pendulum of a clock: each movement extends equally to either side, takes as long, and lasts as long. In jerk nystagmus, the movement in one direction is slow, but the movement in the opposite direction is rapid. In spasmus nutans, the movements of the two eyes do not occur together, but are dissociated. See Table 11-6 for classifications of nystagmus.

Table 11-6

Classi cations of Nystagmus

I. Normal physiologic

  A. End-point
  B. Induced
    1. Drugs
    2. Optokinetic
    3. Caloric
    4. Rotational

II. Congenital

  A. Motor (idiopathic)
  B. Sensory (defective vision)
  C. Latent

III. Acquired

  A. Convergence retraction
  B. Cerebellar
    1. Opsoclonus
    2. Flutter
    3. Dysmetria
  C. Gaze-paretic
  D. Vestibular
    1. Rotary
    2. Horizontal
    3. Vertical
  E. Spasmus nutans
  F. Muscle-paretic
  G. See-saw
  H. Periodic alternating

(Adapted from Cassin B, ed. *Fundamentals for Ophthalmic Technical Personnel.* Philadelphia, Pa: WB Saunders; 1995.)

43. b) Latent nystagmus is a variation of congenital nystagmus that becomes evident only if one eye is covered. The other three can be invoked in a normal patient. End point nystagmus is also called end-gaze and gaze-evoked nystagmus, and sometimes appears when the patient moves the eyes out of primary position. Optokinetic nystagmus is the movements made by the eyes as the patient watches repeating targets, such as fence posts when riding along in the car. (The movement to watch the first object until it passes is known as a *pursuit movement*; the motion to take up fixation on the next object is a *saccade*.) Stimulating the semicircular canals by irrigating the inner ear with warm or cold water also evokes a jerk-type nystagmus. The fast component of the jerk moves to the opposite side of irrigation if cold water is used, but toward the same side of irrigation if warm water is used.

44. b) Oscillopsia is where objects of regard seem to move, jerk, or wiggle when the patient concentrates on them. This phenomenon occurs only in acquired nystagmus; patients with congenital nystagmus do not have this symptom.

45. c) In some cases (notably spasmus nutans), the nystagmus will resolve as the child grows; however, that is not the case with most types of nystagmus. The other statements are true. The head position is adopted in order to move the eyes into a position where the jerking is quieter or stopped, giving the patient clearer vision. The patient "finds" this position (which varies from patient to patient) at an early age, generally when beginning to sit up or stand.

46. d) Cassin, McDavid, and Shamis note that "the underlying defect appears to be disturbed feedback to the gaze centers in the brain stem that interferes with control of the fixation mechanism."

47. a) The tonus, or continued contraction/balancing, of the EOMs maintains the eyes in the "anatomic position of rest" (Burian and von Noorden). Proximal convergence occurs when one becomes aware of an object at near. Accommodative convergence occurs when one focuses on a near object. Fusional convergence is "the fine adjustment of the visual axes, necessary for binocular fixation" (Burian and von Noorden).

48. c) This one might have been tough because of Answers a and b. However, most authors agree that one cannot willfully spread the eyes apart; divergence occurs when convergence is relaxed. If you missed this one, don't worry; the real exam isn't tricky like this. (By the way, divergence is stronger at distance; convergence is stronger at near.)

49. c) The image of the object of regard is falling on corresponding retinal points and appears single. Anything closer or farther than the object of regard appears double (if fixation is maintained) because that image is not falling on corresponding points.

50. d) All of the statements are true. See also Figure 11-3.

51. c) Physiologic diplopia occurs only outside Panum's area, a small area in front of and behind the horopter (see Figure 11-3).

52. b) The size of Panum's area increases as you move outward. This phenomenon is related to retinal structure.

53. b) Burian and von Noorden write that this is due to our "ability to exclude selectively certain unwanted visual impulses from entering consciousness . . . "

54. d) The items in Answers a through c, along with retinal correspondence, are required elements in order for binocular vision to exist. By "similar retinal images," we are referring to similar in size, shape, color, and intensity between the two eyes, since the images must be very similar in order to be fused into one image in the brain.

55. b) For each point on the retina of one eye, there is a corresponding point on the retina of the other eye. As McKenney explains, "corresponding retinal points are elements of both retinas which, when stimulated, give rise to one and the same visual impression." Some (Hoffman) refer to normal retinal correspondence as "harmonious retinal correspondence."

56. b) If normally non-corresponding retinal points "learn" to correspond, the situation is known as abnormal or anomalous retinal correspondence (ARC). This generally occurs in young children with manifest monocular strabismus (most frequently esotropia, says McKenney). The brain develops a "correspondence" between retinal points that would not normally correspond if the eyes were orthophoric.

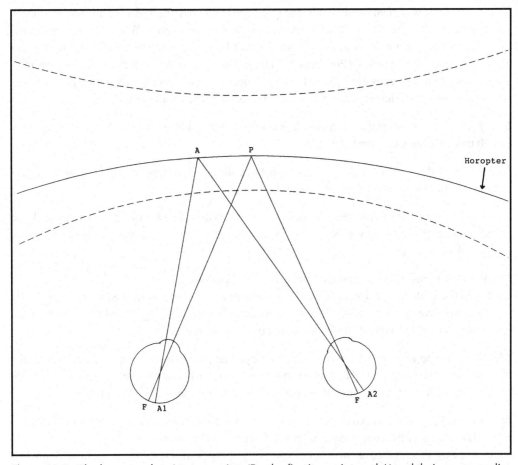

Figure 11-3. The horopter showing two points (P—the fixation point, and A) and their corresponding retinal points in each eye (F—the fovea, A1 and A2). Panum's fusional space lies between the dotted lines. (Reprinted with permission from Lens A, Langley T, Nemeth S, Shea C. *Ocular Anatomy and Physiology*. Thorofare, NJ: SLACK Incorporated; 1998.)

57. a) Fine stereopsis is lacking in the patient with ARC; ARC is not a replacement for normal binocular vision. McKenney calls it "a primitive form of binocular vision." It is important that ARC be prevented early while the visual system is still malleable (eg, by strabismus repair and/or occlusion therapy), because it is not responsive to treatment once established.

58. a) In exotropia associated with convergence insufficiency, one finds that the deviation is greater at near (by 10 prism diopters or more according to Raab; 15 prism diopters or more according to Burian and von Noorden).

59. d) Answers a, b, and c are just the *opposite* of what you would expect. The real symptoms are headaches after near work, letters on the page swimming or jumping, losing their place when reading, closing one eye when reading, double vision at near, and/or falling asleep soon after starting to read. All activities at near require convergence, which is insufficient in this patient's case. Also worth noting: Some of these patients start out with an exodeviation of some kind. Symptoms may occur at any age. Exercises work well as therapy. Hansen says that using base in prism may feel good to the patient, but allows him or her to use even less convergence, further weakening the ability to converge.

60. a) This topic was mentioned in only one reference that I could find (Burian and von Noorden). They state that the AC/A in these patients is low or even zero. While "pencil push-ups" or other such orthoptic exercises probably won't help, they suggest treatment with reading glasses and base-in prism. (Presumably, Hansen would disagree with the base-in prism idea, see Question 59.) They also suggest getting a near point of accommodation on patients with convergence insufficiency prior to treating the convergence insufficiency.

61. c) In exotropia associated with divergence excess, one finds that the deviation is greater (by 10 prism diopters or more) at distance.

62. a) If the difference between the near and distance deviation disappears with a +3.00 add, then the situation is a pseudo-divergence excess.

63. c) A sudden onset of divergence insufficiency is often associated with a preexisting esophoria at distance (Burian and von Noorden). A divergence paralysis is associated with trauma or neurological disease.

64. d) Base out prism in the amount required to give comfortable, single vision at distance is the initial line of therapy. Burian and von Noorden state that the amount of prism may be gradually decreased over a period of weeks or months until they are no longer needed. A bilateral LR resection might be considered if prism therapy does not help.

65. b) When you remove the cover, each/either eye makes a slow movement downward to the midline; thus the eye(s) had drifted up under the cover. Parks and Mitchell recommend holding the cover about 25 cm in front of the patient's eye so you can see what's going on.

66. a) Actually, prolonged occlusion may cause the deviation to *increase*. A few more tidbits:
    The eye under the cover may exhibit pendular, vertical movements
    The eye under the cover may rotate out (excycloduction), exhibiting incycloduction when the cover is removed and the eye returns to the midline
    Not only might the deviation be unequal between the two eyes, it may occur in one eye and not the other.

67. b) Because the occluded eye drifts *up* under the cover (irregardless of which eye is covered), the red image appears to be lower than the fixation light. This is key in differentiating DVD from other cyclovertical abnormalities.

68. d) Burian and von Noorden reported seeing more DVD in children than adults, leading them to state "... we are under the impression that this disorder tends to improve with time." Various theories have been put forth to explain the phenomenon, but Burian and von Noorden state "... it would seem that the innervation association between the eyes ... becomes temporarily suspended ..." It can be differentiated from overaction of the IOs by the red filter/glass test (see Question 67).

69. a) In Graves' disease, strabismus is generally caused by restriction of movement, most often affecting the inferior and/or medical rectus muscles. Forced ductions, in this case, will show "positive for restriction"; that is, you will not be able to move the eye.

70. c) Although there are three types of Duane syndrome, the signs noted in the Question are found in all of them. Hansen (who has wonderful tables on various syndromes and systemic diseases

causing strabismus in her book) says that Duane syndrome "... is thought to be caused by a misfiring, or true co-firing, of the medial rectus and lateral rectus." She further notes that the syndrome occurs mostly in females, and usually in the left eye.

71. b) In Brown syndrome, the superior oblique cannot pass smoothly through the trochlea when the eye is elevated in ADduction. This mimics a weakness of the inferior oblique. Placing the head in a chin-up position puts the eyes into down-gaze, where fusion is possible. Other Notes: Amblyopia rarely occurs in Brown syndrome. Forced ductions are positive. The patient may be ortho in primary gaze.

72. a) In a "regular" third nerve palsy, the pupil of the affected side will almost always be dilated. In a diabetic third nerve palsy, the pupil will be "spared" (ie, not dilated).

73. b) In monofixation syndrome, the patient is frequently anisometropic. All of the other statements are true. The deviation initially appears to be 8 prism diopters or less, but if stressed by prism and alternate cover testing, it will increase (up to 20 prism diopters, says Cassin in *Classification and Characteristics of Eso Deviations*). Hansen says that the associated amblyopia is mild (maybe as little as a half-line of difference); Cassin (in *Classification and Characteristics of Eso Deviations*) states that the amblyopia is usually moderate (20/40 to 20/60) but may extend up to 20/200. She also asserts that monofixation syndrome may be the "end result of strabismus management."

Chapter 7. Advanced Photography

1. b) Luminescence occurs when a suitable material is exposed to incidental light. This causes the electrons (orbiting atomic particles) to jump to different orbits. When the electrons later fall back into their original orbits, a photon of light is given off.

2. d) Fluorescence is a type of luminescence where the excited material glows only while stimulated with the exciting light. (If it lasts for a long time, it is called phosphorescence.)

3. a) Properly excited fluorescein absorbs light in the 465 to 490 nm wavelength range (blue light) and emits light in the 520 to 530 nm range (yellow-green light). This property holds true even when the fluorescein is mixed into the bloodstream.

4. a) Fluorescein angiography is a diagnostic test that provides information about the patient's internal vasculature that is not available any other way.

5. d) The blue exciter filter emits the light that excites the fluorescein. When the dye absorbs the blue light, it is pushed to a higher wavelength and emits yellow-green light.

6. a) The yellow barrier filter acts to block out the blue light of the exciter filter so that the fluorescence will be picked up by the film. It is not used for the red-free photo, but is still needed during the late phase.

7. c) A control photo is taken with both filters in place before the fluorescein is injected. If there is retinal detail on this photograph, it may mean that the exciter filter has aged. Details that are present on the control photo which are due to worn-out filters is termed pseudofluorescence. This phenomenon may also be due to mismatched filters. Another entity that can cause detail

on a control photo is autofluorescence, which is the fluorescence produced by certain ocular conditions, and has nothing to do with the condition of the filters.

8. d) The exciter and barrier filters are matched in order to maximize the fluorescent effect on film. If you mix filter types, you may get filters that overlap, resulting in less than optimum images.

9. a) The pupils need to be well dilated prior to the control photos. In addition, the control photos (see Question 7) must be taken before the dye is introduced. The timer is started at the same time that the dye is pushed.

10. b) The green filter is used to create a "red-free" photo of the fundus. This filter makes the blood vessels appear black, increasing the contrast and making the vessels more visible. The photo provides a reference photo to compare to the angiogram. (This is especially useful if the person interpreting the angiogram does not have access to the patient's records.)

11. a) To quote Cunningham (see Bibliography), "Fluorescein angiography is an invasive procedure with potentially serious side effects." It is imperative that the patient be advised about risks, complications, and side effects. A written consent must be obtained.

12. d) The patient should be informed that the skin and urine may be discolored for several hours after injection. Side effects of the dye can include nausea and vomiting (always have an emesis basin available). Infiltration (extravasation) occurs if the dye is injected into the tissues instead of into the vein. Allergic reaction (including rash, itching, shortness of breath, and anaphylaxis) can also occur, so it is essential to have a properly equipped crash cart handy.

13. b) The photographer needs to be the one to say when the injection should start. If the dye is pushed and the photographer is unaware of it, valuable photographs will be missed in the sequence. In addition, the timer on the camera is started when the dye is pushed.

14. a) A fast b&w film is needed, because the amount of fluorescence emitted by the back of the eye is small.

15. b) If the dye is pushed rapidly into the arm or hand, the dye should appear in the retinal vasculature in about 10 to 20 seconds.

16. capillary phase-3, full venous flow-5, choroidal flush-1, late phase-6, arterial phase-2, early venous phase with laminar flow-4.

17. a) Figure 7-2, b) Figure 7-4, c) Figure 7-3, d) Figure 7-1.

18. c) After the full venous phase (about 24 seconds after injection), the dye slowly moves out of the eye. The "late shots" are taken about 10 minutes after the dye was injected and includes photos of both eyes. Late shots on certain patients may be taken as late as 30 minutes after the injection.

19. d) Extra fluorescein will show up in areas of a leak. (The prefix "hyper" = over, so there is dye over the usual amount.)

20. d) In the case of a blockage in a retinal blood vessel, the dye will be blocked from entering (a filling defect) and hypofluorescence will occur. (The prefix "hypo" = under, so there is dye under the usual amount.)

Table 11-7
Slit Lamp Illumination

Illumination Technique	Mnemonic	Photography Suggestions
Diffuse		overall view of eye; orientation photo
Direct		illumination shown directly on area of interest
Beam	Beagles	narrow beam to localize areas of cornea, broad beam to show extent of affected area
Tangential	take	emphasizes contours and surface texture
Pinpoint	pills	illuminates cell and flare in anterior chamber sparingly.
Specular reflection		
Indirect		area of interest illuminated by reflected light
Proximal	Precise	highlights detail, depth, and density of iris, lens, and corneal lesions
Sclerotic scatter	scientists	corneal changes
Retroillumination	receive	lesions of the cornea, lens, and iris
Transillumination	training.	iris defects

Note: For how-to's on various types of slit lamp illumination, please refer to Series titles *The Slit Lamp Primer* and *Clinical Ocular Photography*.
There are three basic slit lamp illuminations: diffuse, direct, and indirect. The last two have divisions of their own. Each technique is useful in slit lamp photography.

21. a) Hypofluorescence can also occur if the view of the underlying retina is obscured, usually by blood in the vitreous.

22. b) If there is an area where the pigment in the RPE is decreased (a "window"), the normal fluorescence of the choroid is allowed to shine through. This appears in the early phase photos and fades during the late phase (in contrast to an area of hyperfluorescence).

23. d) Before photographing pathology, take a photo of the entire eye using diffuse lighting. This helps orient the viewer when photos are examined later, as well as provides documentation. (It is very difficult to identify a patient, however, from a shot of a single eye.)

24. b) Illumination for slit lamp photos is usually directed from the temporal side. This convention helps orient the viewer, for one thing. For another, it avoids the physical limitations of the patient's nose when positioning the illuminator.

25. a) In tangential illumination, the light source is angled at the eye. This emphasizes the contours of structures, using shadow to show contrast. For further study, see Table 11-7.

26. d) Retroillumination would use light reflected off of the retina to illuminate the lens from behind. This would outline the spokes of the cataract.

27. b) Color slide film is the standard for slit lamp photography. Because the flash and film type are interrelated, the film speed should be chosen according to the output of the light source. Coppinger says that if your flash has a high output, choose a lower ISO film (64 to 200). If the flash has a lower output, choose a film with a higher ISO (200 to 400). Cunningham reminds us that if the photos are for use in a publication that does not use color, b&w film may be appropriate.

28. c) External photography generally includes one head shot for orientation and documentation. A strabismus series would then involve shots showing just the two eyes in the nine positions of gaze. (External photos for ptosis or plastics would include a head shot, then both eyes in primary position, upgaze, and downgaze.)

29. d) If the patient can be identified from the picture, a written consent is needed before displaying or publishing the photo. Verbal consent is not enough. If only the eyes appear in the photo (ie, the patient cannot be identified), the consent is not needed.

30. b) The bilateral view is usually 1:4. The full head shot is 1:10, the orbital shot is 1:3, and the life-size monocular shot is 1:1. (1:7 was a totally bogus answer.)

31. a) The 105 mm lens, with its longer focal length, will increase the camera-to-subject distance. This offers a less intrusive distance for the patient, as well as increases the control over lighting and cornea reflections for the photographer. (This is in contrast to the "normal" working lens of 50 mm, which requires that the camera be closer to the subject.)

32. b) The point is to avoid obscuring pathology with the flash reflection. The smallest reflector available should be used. A point source is better than a ring flash, especially if it is mounted on an adjustable bracket so it can be rotated.

33. b) The specular microscope was developed specifically to evaluate the layer of cells making up the corneal endothelium. (It is very difficult, although possible, to see this layer with the slit lamp.)

34. d) Because of the high magnification used, even a tiny movement of the eye sends the view of the cells swooshing across the eyepiece or monitor. Video film is used to tape the viewing session, then individual frames are projected and examined later. Individual photographs (usually on an instantty of film) can then be created from a single video frame.

35. d) Any of the listed methods may be used. A grid may be laid over the viewing screen. The cells within the boundaries are counted, as well as the cells touching one vertical and one horizontal line of the square. This number is then multiplied by a constant. (Check the user's manual to find the constant for a particular instrument and a specific grid.) Some instruments provide a computer print out. Other manufacturers supply template cards which are pictures of cells. You compare the patient's display to the cards and select the best match.

36. c) Changing the silver halides to metallic silver "develops" the latent image on the film.

37. d) The stop bath is used to "stop" the action of the developer.

38. d) The film must be protected from light until it has been through the fixer, which removes any unexposed silver from the film. Activities in Answers a through c occur prior to fixing.

39. c) Tapping the tank (prior to immersing the film) will loosen any bubbles clinging to the tank's side which could ultimately wind up on the film. Tiny areas of film that are covered by a bubble will not be exposed to the developing fluid.

40. a) Diluting the developer with water 1:1 is a great way to prepare a developer of the proper temperature. However, changing the developing time is then necessary. It is not simply a matter of doubling the developing time; you will have to check the manufacturer's recommendations to see how much longer to develop. Another drawback is that the diluted developer may not

be reused, which is sometimes possible if the developer is left full-strength. (*Note*: When full-strength developer is reused, it is also necessary to add developing time as the solution is exhausted.)

41. a) The developing tank must be agitated when developing the film. The tank (if not equipped with a stirring rod) may be swirled with a circular motion or inverted. Cunningham notes that some solution manufacturers give specific directions for agitation. Coppinger says that the important thing is to be consistent with your time intervals. The film should not be exposed to light at this point.

Chapter 8. Advanced Pharmacology

1. b) The stability of the drug refers to its ability to stay in an active form with a shelf-life long enough to withstand reasonable storage after manufacturing and distribution.

2. d) Light, moisture, and heat may each have an effect on a drug, causing stability to be reduced. Light-sensitive materials are generally dispensed in opaque packages. High or low humidity may also affect medication, so packages should always remain sealed until used, and bottles should be tightly capped. Excessive heat may also reduce the stability of the drug. (Remind patients not to leave their medicines in the glove compartment of their car, which can get as hot as an oven in the summer.) Extreme cold and/or freezing may also cause the drug to degrade. Most medications are best stored at room temperature.

3. c) Oxygen can decrease the stability of a drug, once the package is opened and the medication is exposed. Antioxidants (such as sodium bisulfate) are added to a solution to help prevent oxidation.

4. c) According to Duvall and Kershner, a solution that is slightly acidic tends to be more stable.

5. c) Tolerance is the quality of the drug to be "tolerated" by the eye by not causing any ill effects to the eye's tissues. The pH of a drug affects, in part, the amount of ocular irritation that occurs on installation. (See also Question 6.)

6. a) Acids have a pH below 7 and alkalines have a pH over 7. A pH of 7 is neutral. The pH of the tear film is about 7.4. Solutions with a pH between 6.6 and 7.8 are generally well tolerated. Outside these boundaries stinging becomes a problem.

7. b) Buffers are chemicals that are added to the medication to put the pH into the tolerated range between 6 and 8. This is not always a solution to the pH problem, however, because some medications become less stable if the pH is too alkaline. The solubility of the drug may be adversely affected as well.

8. a) Tonicity refers to the concentration of a drug in regard to the osmotic balance on and in the eye. Osmosis refers to the process where the fluid in a solution moves across a membrane from the area of low chemical concentration to the area of high chemical concentration in an effort to equalize the concentration of the chemical on both sides of the membrane. A solution with a high chemical (drug) concentration would be hypertonic ("hyper" = over). A solution with a low drug concentration is hypotonic ("hypo" = under). If two solutions have the same tonicity, they are said to be isotonic ("iso" = same).

9. c) See also Question 8. The tonicity of the tear film is 0.9% sodium chloride. Medications that fall into a tonicity range between 0.6 to 1.8 are generally well tolerated by the eye. Buffer chemicals (such as glycerin, sodium, and potassium chloride) are sometimes added to a drug to place its tonicity within the ideal range.

10. d) A hypertonic drug has a chemical (drug) concentration high enough to cause fluid to move out of the tissues of the eye in an effort to equalize the concentration. Thus, hypertonic drugs may be used topically to reduce corneal edema (as in 5% sodium chloride drops or ointment).

11. b) Oral glycerin is used as a hypertonic drug given to quickly reduce the volume of aqueous in an angle-closure glaucoma attack. (*Study Note*: Hypertonic is sometimes also referred to as hyperosmolar.) Mannitol and urea, also hypertonic drugs, are given intravenously.

12. a) While the drug may be uncontaminated (ie, no bacteria or other organisms have gotten into it), it is no longer considered sterile once opened.

13. c) Preservatives are added to inhibit or kill organisms that may contaminate the medication.

14. a) There are two classes of preservatives: bacteriostatic (which inhibit cell growth) and bacteriocidal (which kill the cell or prevent its reproduction).

15. b) Bensalkonium chloride is a popular bacteriostatic preservative in current use. Thimerosal, a mercuric bacteriostatic preservative, is not as widely used any more because of the number of patients who develop an allergic sensitivity to the chemical after only a short exposure.

16. d) A side effect is an effect that the drug has on the body other than the desired or intended effect. Tingling in the extremities while taking acetazolamide is an example of this. Other examples include gastrointestinal disturbances (beta blockers and others), brow ache (pilocarpine), or elevated intraocular pressure (steroids). An allergy, however, is an immune response when an individual becomes sensitized to an antigen. The classic example is a rash. Anaphylactic shock, which is a severe allergic reaction, can include difficulty with breathing and a pulse that is fast and weak. It can become so severe as to lead to death.

17. a) A local allergic reaction to a topical ocular medication can include rash (of eyelids), itching, redness (conjunctival and lids), and swelling (conjunctival and lids).

18. a) A localized reaction is limited to one area, generally the area of drug administration. In the eye, this would usually be evidenced by redness, chemosis, watering, and itching. Irrigation is the first aid action you should take. It is also important to note the allergy in the patient's chart so that the drug is avoided in the future. The items in Answer c apply to anaphylactic shock and would be administered by the physician.

19. d) All of the answers list possible scenarios for an abnormal drug reaction. In addition to patients whose general health is compromised, the action of a drug may also not be what is anticipated if the patient is very old or very young. If more than one drug is being used, the medications may interact with one another. This could cause a chemical reaction, or it could accent or decrease the effect of one or both drugs. Some drugs can have a toxic effect on the body. An example is the effect of chloroquine on the retinal cones. Finally, a chemical reaction could cause toxicity, unexpected interactions, or other effects (such as forming deposits in tissues).

20. d) Blocking off the puncta prevents the drug from traveling through the nasolacrimal system and into the throat, where it can be swallowed. Punctal occlusion is accomplished by gently pressing the fingers into the nasal corners of the closed eyes.

21. d) The "fight or flight" response (including all the details listed) results from stimulation to the sympathetic branch of the autonomic nervous system. By way of review, the autonomic nervous system controls "automatic" functions such as pulse and respiration rates, blood flow, digestion, etc.

22. b) The other branch of the autonomic nervous system is the parasympathetic system. It has essentially the opposite effect of the sympathetic system. (You should especially note that pupil constriction is a product of the parasympathetic system.)

23. b) A neurotransmitter is a biochemical released by the neurons (nerve cells) that take a message of action or inaction to the target organ or tissue. Once a neurotransmitter is released, it attaches itself to specific receptor sites. When the neurotransmitter is connected to a receptor (which might be in the heart, organs, glands, or blood vessels), then the specific action is carried out. (You might think of this as a key that fits into a lock.) The neurotransmitters for the sympathetic nervous system are epinephrine (also called adrenaline) and norepinephrine. Drugs that have their effect on the sympathetic system are also known as adrenergic drugs. (*Study Note*: "adren" appears in adrenaline and adrenergic.) The sympathetic system has several types of receptors: alpha and beta. You will sometimes see drugs listed as alpha or beta blockers; this is a reference to the specific types of receptors of the sympathetic system.

24. d) Acetylcholine is the major neurotransmitter of the parasympathetic system. Thus, a cholinergic drug affects the parasympathetic system. It is especially important to understand that the drugs in these two groups are classified according to the system that they affect, and not by the effects they have on the body. Please refer to Table 11-8 as you go through this set of Questions.

25. a) Something that copies could also be said to mime. The word mime is your clue to help you remember that sympathomimetic drugs mime, copy, or imitate the sympathetic system.

26. d) Phenylephrine, used for pupil mydriasis, is sympathomimetic. It mimics the sympathetic response of pupil dilation by causing the iris dilator muscle to contract. It has no effect on the ciliary muscle, so accommodation is not affected. Please refer to Table 11-9 for more study information on adrenergic (sympathetic) and cholinergic (parasympathetic) drugs as you answer the remaining questions.

27. b) Vasoconstriction is an effect of the sympathetic system. Thus these sympathomimetic drugs (in addition to phenylephrine and oxymetazoline) are used to whiten the eye.

28. a) Apraclonidine and brimonidine act to decrease aqueous formation by assisting specific receptor sites (alpha receptors) in the sympathetic system. Thus they are sympathomime.

29. d) A sympatholytic drug blocks the pathway required for a response in the sympathetic system. (*Study Note*: The word "lysis" means to destroy something. A sympatholytic drug "destroys" the effect of the sympathetic system.)

30. d) Beta blockers (which include timolol, betaxolol, levobunolol, carteolol, and metipranolol) are sympatholytic agents used to decrease the formation of aqueous. Their action is on the sympathetic system (they block the beta receptors in the sympathetic system), so they are adrenergic drugs.

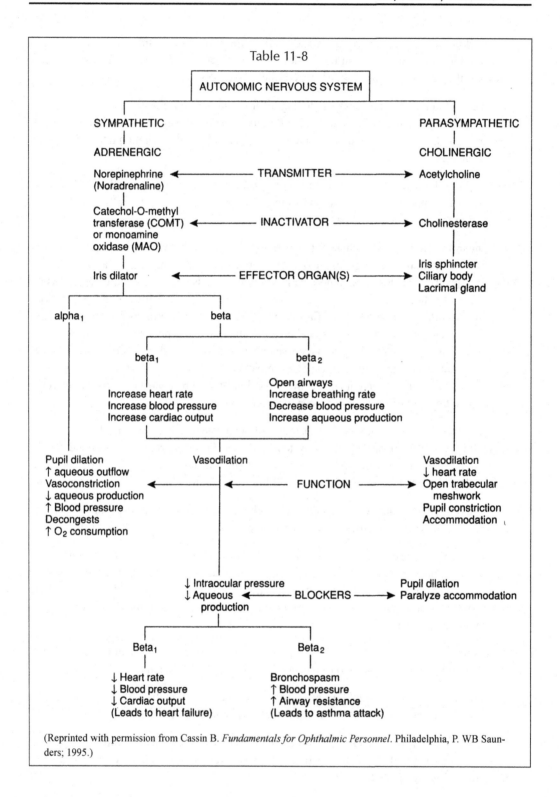

Table 11-8

AUTONOMIC NERVOUS SYSTEM

SYMPATHETIC | PARASYMPATHETIC

ADRENERGIC | CHOLINERGIC

Norepinephrine ◄———— TRANSMITTER ————► Acetylcholine
(Noradrenaline)

Catechol-O-methyl
transferase (COMT) ◄———— INACTIVATOR ————► Cholinesterase
or monoamine
oxidase (MAO)

Iris sphincter
Iris dilator ◄———— EFFECTOR ORGAN(S) ————► Ciliary body
Lacrimal gland

alpha$_1$ beta

beta$_1$ beta$_2$

Increase heart rate   Open airways
Increase blood pressure   Increase breathing rate
Increase cardiac output   Decrease blood pressure
    Increase aqueous production

Pupil dilation   Vasodilation   Vasodilation
↑ aqueous outflow   ↓ heart rate
Vasoconstriction ◄——— ◄——— FUNCTION ————► Open trabecular
↓ aqueous production   meshwork
↑ Blood pressure   Pupil constriction
Decongests   Accommodation
↑ O$_2$ consumption

↓ Intraocular pressure   Pupil dilation
↓ Aqueous ◄——— BLOCKERS ————► Paralyze accommodation
production

Beta$_1$ Beta$_2$

↓ Heart rate   Bronchospasm
↓ Blood pressure   ↑ Blood pressure
↓ Cardiac output   ↑ Airway resistance
(Leads to heart failure)   (Leads to asthma attack)

(Reprinted with permission from Cassin B. *Fundamentals for Ophthalmic Personnel.* Philadelphia, P. WB Saunders; 1995.)

Table 11-9
Drug Categories

I. Adrenergic drugs (sympathetic system)

A. Mydriatics (sympathomimetics)
phenylephrine
hydroxyamphetamine
cocaine

B. Decrease aqueous formation
  1. Sympathomimetics (alpha receptor agonists)
    apraclonidine
    brimonidine
  2. Sympatholytics (beta receptor blockers/antagonists)
    betaxolol
    levobunolol
    metipranolol
    timolol
    carteolol

C. Increase aqueous outflow (sympathomimetics)
epinephrine
dipivefrin

D. Vasoconstrictors (sympathomimetics)
phenylephrine
naphazoline
oxymetazoline
tetrahydrozoline

E. Dilation reversal (sympatholytic)
dapiprazole
thymoxamine

II. Cholinergic drugs (parasympathetic system)

A. Miotics (parasympathomimetics)
  1. Direct-acting
    pilocarpine
    carbachol
  2. Indirect-acting (cholinesterase inhibitors)
    physostigmine
    echothiophate
    isoflurophate
    demarcarium bromide

B. Cycloplegics (parasympatholytics)
atropine
scopalomine (hyoscine)
homatropine
cyclopentolate
tropicamide

C. Diagnostic (cholinesterase inhibitor)
edrophonium

D. Muscle paralysis (parasympatholytic)
botulinum A toxin

31. b) The drugs dapiprazole and thymoxamine are sympatholytic drugs that are adrenergic (sympathetic) blockers (they block the alpha receptors). Thus they can be used to reverse mydriasis.

32. c) Pilocarpine, which is used to control glaucoma, is a parasympathomimetic drug. In other words, it mimics the action of the parasympathetic system and causes pupillary miosis. All of the miotics are parasympathetic agonists (agonists are good guys who want to help!). There are two groups of miotics: direct acting (pilocarpine and carbachol), which act directly on the end-organ, and indirect acting. The indirect-acting miotics are cholinesterase inhibitors, which are explained in Questions 38 through 41.

33. a) The parasympathomimetics cause the iris sphincter and ciliary body to contract. This pulls on the scleral spur, which opens up the trabecular meshwork and increases the outflow of aqueous.

34. d) Accommodative spasms, associated with the parasympathomimetics, can cause a brow ache when the patient first begins using them. This tends to decrease with time.

35. b) This question was packed with info! First, if the drug is cholinergic-blocking, this is telling you that acetylcholine (the neurotransmitter for the parasympathetic system) has been blocked. Thus, the parasympathetic effect has been destroyed or lysed (parasympatholytic). This dilates the pupil and freezes accommodation.

36. b) Botulinum A toxin is a parasympatholytic drug that blocks acetylcholine and has the effect of paralyzing muscles. In tiny amounts, it can be used to treat blepharospasm if injected into the eyelid muscles, or to treat strabismus if injected into the proper extraocular muscle.

37. b) The cycloplegics act to block acetylcholine from acting on the muscles. This paralyzes the iris sphincter and ciliary muscle, resulting in dilation and loss of accommodation. The cycloplegics include atropine, scopalomine (hyoscine), homatropine, cyclopentolate, and tropicamide.

38. a) Cholinesterase is a biochemical that act as a "clean up man" for acetylcholine. Once a neurotransmitter is released, it attaches itself to specific receptor sites. When the neurotransmitter is connected to a receptor (which might be in the heart, organs, glands, or blood vessels), then the specific action is carried out. (You might think of this as a key that fits into a lock.) Cholinesterase removes acetylcholine from the receptor sites. This has the effect of reducing the parasympathetic effect.

39. d) Cholinesterase removes acetylcholine from the receptor sites. This has the effect of reducing the parasympathetic reaction. If you are inhibiting cholinesterase, then you are allowing acetylcholine to accumulate. This has the effect of a continued stimulation of the parasympathetic system. (Note: There is an error in the Duvall/Kershner book that says cholinesterase inhibitors have a sympathetic effect. They actually enhance the parasympathetic effect.)

40. b) The indirect-acting miotics exert their effect by blocking cholinesterase, thus allowing acetylcholine to act freely. These miotics include physostigmine, echothiophate, isoflurophate, and demecarium bromide.

41. b) Edrophonium (or Tensilon, ICN Pharmaceuticals, Costa Mesa, Calif) is a cholinesterase inhibitor (also known as anticholinesterase drug) used to differentiate ptosis due to myasthenia gravis from that due to other causes. (If the ptosis is due to myasthenia, an IV injection of edrophonium will cause a temporary elevation of the lid.)

Chapter 9. Special Instruments and Techniques

1. b) The word "laser" is an acronym for light amplification by stimulated emission of radiation. The electrons are provided by a chemical substance (eg, argon gas or yttrium-aluminum-garnet [YAG] crystal). The electrons are "pumped up" by exposing them to a power source such as heat or electricity and are thus excited to such a state that they emit photons of monochromatic light. (Monochromatic meaning single wavelength.) The wavelength, direction, and phase of the photons are all the same. This produces a narrow column of light that is extremely intense.

2. a) The argon and krypton lasers are absorbed by tissues containing hemoglobin. The absorbed laser light is transformed into thermal (heat) energy, and coagulation occurs. (To get a mental image of this, it can be compared to welding.) See Table 11-10 for a summary of laser types, actions, and uses.

3. d) Because argon laser light is absorbed by hemoglobin, this laser is wonderfully suited for treating disorders of the blood vessels, such as diabetic retinopathy (both leaking vessels and neovascularization) and vein occlusions. It is also used to treat some retinal detachments (if they are localized and there is no traction) and retinal holes. Its spot size is too large to treat the macula.

4. a) Fluorescein will absorb the 488 nm wavelengths . . . those of the argon laser. Thus fluorescein dye should be irrigated from the eye prior to the procedure.

5. a) In order to increase drainage after trabeculectomy, the scleral flap sutures can be lysed by focusing the krypton (or argon) laser right through the conjunctiva.

6. d) The krypton laser is not absorbed by retinal blood vessels (so it passes through hemorrhages), but it is absorbed by melanin (present in the choroid and RPE). Therefore it is ideal for the structures listed. (It also passes easily through cataracts.)

7. b) The ionizing (Q-charged) YAG laser results in the ionization of tissue from high heat plus mechanical and acoustic shock waves. This produces a "microexplosion" (or photodisruption) that destroys the tissue. (It is important to note that the heat itself does not ablate the tissue, but rather the "explosion.")

8. d) The photodisruptive power of the YAG laser makes it ideal for punching a hole through the iris. Probably the more common use, however, is laser capsulotomy following cataract surgery.

9. b) The excimer laser (excited dimer) destroys tissue by using short-pulsed ultraviolet radiation with a short wavelength.

10. a) A thin area of corneal stroma can be ablated by the excimer laser to flatten the corneal cap during a refractive procedure known as photorefractive keratotomy, or PRK. The excimer is also used to remove corneal scars.

11. c) Tissues with a high water content are treated with the carbon dioxide laser because water absorbs the laser light.

Table 11-10
Lasers in Ophthalmology

Laser	Wavelength	Action	Uses
I. Thermal			
Argon	blue-green (488 to 515 nm) low energy continuous wave	photocoagulation absorbed by hemoglobin, melanin, and xanthophil	retinal vascular disease choroidal neovascularization trabeculoplasty iridotomy suture lysis
Krypton	red (647 nm) continuous wave	photocoagulation absorbed by melanin, to a lesser degree by hemoglobin (not absorbed by retinal vessels) and xanthophil passes more readily through lens opacities and vitreous hemorrhages	same as argon but deeper choroid
CO_2	infrared long wavelength low penetration	photovaporization (photo-evaporation) absorbed by water	skin lesions fine, bloodless skin incisions cautery
Tunable dye	adjustable (green to red)	photocoagulation variably absorbed by melanin, hemoglobin, and xanthophil	same as argon and krypton
Diode laser	infrared (805 nm)	photocoagulation sometimes used in conjunction with ICG dye	retinal vascular disease choroidal neovascularization
Frequency-doubled YAG	green (532 nm) continuous wave	photocoagulation	same as krypton
II. Ionizing			
Q-switched YAG	infrared (1064 nm) pulsed laser	photodisruption ("cold, cutting") very tiny spot sizes	incisions/cutting synechiotomy capsulotomy vitreous adhesions iridotomy
III. Photochemical			
Excimer	UV light (photo-evaporation)	photoablation breaks chemical bonds of tissues	corneal opacities refractive surgery
Photodynamic therapy	red-infrared (665 to 732 nm)	causes chemical changes that result in vascular occlusion and cellular disruption used in conjunction with photosensitive agents	malignant tumors choroidal neovascularization

12. b) Skin cells have a very high water content, ideal for treatment with the carbon dioxide laser. The laser produces an extremely fine line, making it useful in making incisions during eyelid surgery. The drawback in using it to remove lesions is that there is no specimen left for biopsy, so it is used mainly if the physician is sure that the growth is not malignant.

13. b) The "tunable" part of a tunable dye laser refers to the ability to select a wavelength (from green to red) that is appropriate to the work being done. (Other lasers have a fixed wavelength which are useful for only specific uses.) The tunable dye laser can be used for iridotomy, iridoplasty, and trabeculoplasty.

14. c) The laser microendoscope combines a light source, laser, and videocamera. It is actually inserted into the eye, and the eye's interior is projected onto a screen. The physician can then visualize the tissue requiring laser treatment. Because an incision is necessary, this type of treatment is often performed during other intraocular surgery, such as cataract removal. The argon laser is used in the microendoscope.

15. c) Cell death occurs when sensitized tissue is exposed to the laser. Red laser light has been used in ophthalmology to treat cancers of the eye tissues.

16. b) Like conventional X-rays, CT uses ionizing radiation. Bone is the most visible on a CT, but the soft tissues also absorb enough radiation to be visible to varying degrees. Instead of producing images on film, the CT images are gathered by electronic radiation detectors and displayed on a monitor. The images may also be printed out.

17. d) Dye may be used during a CT scan in order to provide contrast among the tissues being studied. This works because the dye increases the radiation absorption of certain tissues, making them more visible. (In fact, the order for the scan often reads "CT of head and orbits with and without contrast" if the dye is to be used.)

18. b) The tissue to be examined is exposed to radio waves. When the tissue is bombarded by the radio waves, the atoms give off an electronic signal. (This occurs when, first, the magnetic field aligns hydrogen ions in the tissues. When the magnetic field is turned off, the ions fall back into place, giving off the "signal.") A computer "captures" the signal and displays the image on a monitor. The images may also be printed.

19. c) The CT scan is especially useful for evaluating hard tissue (ie, bone), and would be most useful in this case.

20. a) Because a strong magnetic field is created, any patient with a pacemaker, metal implants, or embedded metal cannot have the test.

21. c) The MRI is especially good for soft tissue evaluation. Solid tissue produces only low-intensity signals on an MRI; soft tissues signals are higher. (The opposite is true of a CT.) A B-scan would give some information on the optic nerve, but could not provide anything as far back as the chiasm.

22. c) Only B-scan ultrasound provides a two-dimensional image of the globe. A-scan provides a one-dimensional measurement.

23. c) "After movement" refers to any "swishing" movement of a structure (usually a membrane or vascularized tumor) which can be observed during the B-scan (not after) when the patient

is asked to move the eye. The term "dynamic" refers to motion. The B-scan offers a real-time opportunity to observe the interior of the eye.

24. a) A vitreous detachment will be more "swishy"; a retinal detachment usually looks stiffer and the movement is not as pronounced.

25. b) If the patient cannot see out, then the physician cannot see in. If the retina is detached, there is little hope of visual improvement despite cataract surgery. If the retina is attached, the physician and patient may consider trying the surgery, hoping for visual improvement.

26. c) The pulse emitter generates the ultrasonic waves into the tissue. The waves that are reflected back are picked up by the receiver and enlarged by the amplifier. The signal processor filters out the "noise" and reshapes the signal, sending them on to some type of display screen.

27. d) The gates (calipers or over-lights) are measuring markers that tell the computer what part of the scan to measure (eg, the vertical or horizontal dimensions of a tumor). On an A-scan for axial length, most instruments have an "automatic" mode where the machine selects the appropriate-appearing spikes and measures those automatically.

28. b) Standardized echography combines standardized A-scan (used to identify characteristics of the tissue), contact B-scan, and specific examination techniques. It is especially useful in differentiating between different types of tumors. The B-scan provides a two-dimensional picture of the tumor, as well as size measurements. The standardized A-scan gives information about the tissue itself (such as is it fluid-filled, how reflective is the tissue, etc).

29. c) This fact is the basis for understanding orientation of B-scan displays. The B-scan probe has a mark on it (usually a white line). No matter which way you hold the probe, the area directly under the white line is always displayed at the top of the screen. This also shows why standardized technique and prompt documentation is necessary . . . no one but the ultrasonographer knows how the probe was oriented on a particular display.

30. Labeling: a) cornea, b) iris, c) lens, d) macula, e) optic nerve.

31. a) Most artifacts in B-scans are caused when the probe does not make complete contact with the eye. This creates an area of reflection which is transmitted to the display. Use lots of gel to help keep good contact. The presence of air inside the eye will cause an artifact, but this is not the cause of "most" artifacts, which is specified by the question.

32. b) The three probe positions are transverse, longitudinal, and axial. These positions are further defined by the location of the probe on the eye. In the axial view, the probe is placed on the center of the cornea and aimed directly at the posterior of the eye with the probe marker at 12:00 (ie, vertical). In this view, the center of the image shows the posterior lens surface and optic nerve.

33. c) Metal is so highly reflective that it bounces all the ultrasound back to the receiver. This casts a "shadow" behind the foreign body.

34. Labeling: a) Figure 9-4, b) Figure 9-2, c) Figure 9-5, d) Figure 9-3.

35. b) The desired postoperative refractive error must be entered into the equation in order for the proper IOL to be selected. In some cases it may be best for a Plano postoperative refraction. However, some patients may prefer to be left a little nearsighted in order to read without correction following surgery. Other possibilities exist as well.

36. d) In the absence of other problems (such as vastly dissimilar K readings between the two eyes), this reading is within the normal range. You were not given enough information to indicate whether or not lenticular astigmatism was present.

37. c) Nearly all of the IOL calculation formulas are based on the same type of equation in which the axial length of the eye, the depth of the anterior chamber, tissue velocity, and the refractive powers of the cornea and IOL are factors.

38. a) The A-constant is a number provided by the IOL manufacturer that is specific to that type of IOL. The number is entered into the IOL calculation formula.

39. c) All are true except evaluating macular degeneration (in situations where the ERG is not sensitive enough to pick it up). Cortical blindness is better evaluated by running a visually evoked potential (VEP); however, one might run an ERG to rule out the retina as a factor in suspected cortical blindness. An ERG might also be used to evaluate chorioretinal degenerations or inflammations, giant-cell arteritis, hypothyroidism, and hypervitaminosis. Finally, ruling out the retina as a problem in dyslexia and disproving visual loss in the hysterical and malingering patient can also be done via ERG.

40. b) The ERG is a test of the entire retina, including rods and cones. The test can also be modified to test rods or cones alone. During the test, the patient is exposed to a flash of light. This causes all the rods and cones to fire at the same time (a mass retinal response). The mass retinal response is recorded and evaluated. There is a specialized ERG known as a focal ERG which tests only a small area of the retina (usually the macula), but this test is not in common use. There is also a pattern ERG used to test the function of the ganglion cells. However, the full-field ERG, described first, is the one generally referred to when one speaks of an ERG. A Ganzfeld globe, which is similar to a Goldmann perimeter in appearance, is used for the test.

41. a) There is a direct correlation between the amplitude of the ERG and retinal function. Thus, if the ERG amplitude is reduced by 50%, then there is a 50% reduction in the function of the retina. (A common cause of this would be a retinal detachment.) The ERG may be non-recordable if less than 10% of the retina is functioning. Van Boemel notes that "there is not a direct correlation between ERGs and visual acuity."

42. c) The active electrode is placed on the eye, on or next to the cornea. The reference electrode is attached to the skin (face, forehead, or lateral canthus). The ground electrode is also a skin electrode (forehead or behind the ear). The ERG wave is created by the active and reference electrodes (it is actually the difference between the two). (It is worth noting that if the electrode is a bipolar electrode such as the Burian-Allen, then both the active and reference electrodes are over the cornea.)

43. d) The patient is dilated with 2.5% phenylephrine and 1% tropicamide, then dark-adapted for 20 minutes (minimum). The test is generally performed in darkroom-like conditions (ie, no light entering under doors, and a red light to allow some vision without disturbing dark adaptation).

44. b) Because seizures can sometimes be triggered by flashing lights, a patient with epilepsy (or other seizure disorder) should be tested with a single flash and fewer times. The light should be covered with a red filter as well so that only cones are stimulated.

45. b) The protocol for an ERG has been standardized by the International Society for the Clinical Electrophysiology of Vision and the National Retinitis Pigmentosa Foundation, Inc. After the

dilated patient is dark-adapted, the red-light (darkroom light) is turned off. The patient is positioned in the Ganzfeld bowl, asked to look at a tiny red fixation light, and to move the eyes as little as possible. The dark-adapted portion of the test starts with the scotopic ERG, a very dim, filtered light that flashes about once every 2 seconds. Next, the process is repeated with an unfiltered light (this is the mesopic part of the test). Still in the dark, the oscillatory potential is obtained by flashing the brightest, unfiltered light (after slightly altering the parameters of the computer for this portion of the examination only). The lights in the room and bowl are now turned on for the light-adapted phase of the test. The individual must be allowed to light adapt for at least 5 minutes prior to starting the second portion of the test. The photopic portion uses a bright, non-filtered light (a single flash or a set of flashes that are averaged). The flicker fusion test is done by flashing the stimulus 30 times per second. (By the way, this is an objective test, requiring no observation or response from the patient.)

46. b) The a-wave is generated by the rods and cones (photoreceptor cells) and the b-wave comes from the mid-retinal layers (containing the Mueller and bipolar cells). The waves are evaluated for amplitude and delay (time from stimulus to peak of b-wave). The cone ERG produces a fast, small waveform that consists of an a-wave and b-wave. The amplitude of the cone b-wave should be about 100 microvolts. The rod ERG produces a slower wave form that shows no real a-wave (at very low light levels) but a very large b-wave. The rod ERG b-wave should be about 200 microvolts in amplitude.

47. d) Slowing of the waves might be seen in *early* retinitis pigmentosa. As the retina degenerates, the waveform becomes slower and lower in amplitude. But at the end-stage point, less than 10% of the retina is functional and the ERG would not be recordable (under most circumstances). The individual's visual fields would be down to about 10 degrees and there would be severe visual impairment. Reduced amplitude of both waves (without any slowing of the waveform) is seen when some portion of the retina is not functioning, but the other portion is normal (as in retinal detachment). The normal a-/abnormal b scenario is seen in situations where the photoreceptors are active but there is some problem in the middle retinal layers.

48. c) The EOG is a test of RPE function used when the physician suspects some type of retinal abnormality (especially degenerative disorders). (The rods also contribute to the EOG, but it is used primarily to test RPE function.) Technically speaking, the EOG measures the "standing electrical potential" between the front and back of the eye. Van Boemel explains this concept by comparing the eye to a battery which runs down in the dark and charges up in the light. She says, "In order for this battery-like effect to occur, a barrier must be present between the two poles (back and the front of the eye). That barrier happens to be the RPE . . . "

49. b) The EOG is a measurement of the electrical activity that occurs between the front (cornea) and back of the eye. The cornea is the positive pole; when the cornea moves toward an electrode (to pick up fixation on the stimulus, which is located far-right or far-left), the electrode becomes positive as well. The eye movement is recorded. The main point of the test, where retinal function is concerned, is to compare the voltage change (seen in differences in eye movement amplitude) in the light- vs dark-adapted state. Remembering our battery analogy, the healthy eye "runs down" in the dark and "re-charges" in the light. Thus there is an increasing amplitude of the eye movement in the EOG read-out in response to light adaptation . . . again, if the eye is healthy. The waves themselves on the EOG are generated by eye movement, but the voltage is created by the cornea-retina potential known as the cornea-fundal potential.

50. d) The patient is dilated to allow for full light adaptation during that portion of the test. There are five skin electrodes. Four active electrodes are placed one at the canthi of each eye. The ground electrode is placed on the forehead. Once dilation has taken effect, the patient is initially light-adapted for a few minutes, then dark-adapted for 2 minutes. At this point the test begins.

51. b) Let's back up for a moment and look at how the test itself is conducted. A Ganzfeld bowl is used, as in the ERG. After 2 minutes of dark adaptation, the test begins. The patient is asked to look at a right and left diode as they alternate lighting up every 2 seconds. The lights alternate for about a 15 to 20 second period, then the patient is asked to close his or her eyes. This process is repeated so that the patient is tested every 2 minutes up to 14 minutes of dark adaptation. The waves and voltages from each of these is recorded. By the time the 14 minutes is up, the "battery" is pretty much worn down. The item of interest here is the smallest amplitude, which is called the *dark trough*. At this point, the light inside the bowl is turned on. The test is repeated after 2 minutes of light adaptation and continues every 2 minutes up to 14. Instead of closing the eyes between sessions, the patient is asked to continue to stare straight ahead to ensure continuing adaptation as the "battery" recharges. This time we are interested in the largest amplitude, known as the *light peak*. The comparison of the light peak to the dark trough is made as a ratio known as the Arden ratio. The Arden ratio is often called the light/dark ratio.

52. c) A normal Arden ratio is 2.0. A ratio that falls below 1.55 is considered abnormal. An abnormal Arden ratio is considered to exist because the junctions between the RPE cells are not tight (ie, broken down by disease) and there is less of a barrier between the two poles of the eye. Van Boemel says that the EOG in end-stage retinitis pigmentosa (where the photoreceptor cells and pigment epithelium are atrophied) will be around 1.00 to 1.30.

53. b) The RPE (as well as the photoreceptor cells) is involved in retinitis pigmentosa. In Best's disease (a juvenile-onset type of macular degeneration), the ERG is normal but the EOG will be abnormal. Retinal toxicities affecting the RPE may be due to medications (or other substances) or intraocular metallic foreign bodies. The EOG is used to evaluate nystagmus and nerve palsies (see Questions 54 and 55), but this would not be a retinal type of EOG evaluation.

54. b) Testing ocular movements with the EOG is not interested in the eye as a "battery." To test horizontal eye movements, the electrodes are placed at the canthi as with a retinal EOG. To test vertical eye movements, the electrodes are placed above the brow and on the lower lid. The patient sits inside a striped drum and told to "watch the stripes" as the drum is rotated. The character of the movement tracings can indicate limited motility and fatigue patterns that may be characteristic of certain muscle and nerve disorders.

55. a) An EOG might be indicated to evaluate a third, fourth, or sixth nerve palsy. The test may also be used in cases of mechanical restriction (as in an orbital floor fracture or severe scarring following strabismus surgery), neurological diseases (such as myasthenia gravis), and Duane's syndrome.

56. c) The VEP is also called the visual evoked response (VER) or the visual evoked cortical potential (VECP). It is the response of the occipital cortex (also called the visual cortex) of the brain to a specific visual stimulus. It "provides excellent information about the functional

integrity of the visual system . . . " (Van Boemel). Unfortunately, it does not tell you which part of the visual system is at fault if an abnormal result is obtained. The VEP *does* let you know whether or not the signal is getting through all the way to the brain, and whether or not it is getting through well, poorly, or not at all. The rods and cones, as well as the ganglion cells and optic nerve, all contribute to the VEP. If there is a total retinal detachment, no electrical signal will be generated by the retina to be delivered to the brain. If the optic nerve is completely damaged by increased IOP, the retinal signal will not get to the brain as a result of the optic nerve damage. In both instances, the VEP would be non-recordable but for reasons other than occipital cortex abnormality.

57. d) For most settings, a flashing light and an alternating checkerboard pattern are used in VEP testing. The sinusoidal gratings are used sometimes in laboratory settings. The light flash test gives information about whether or not the visual system as a whole is intact. The alternating checkerboard is an indicator of visual acuity (the examiner varies the size of the grid). It takes about half a second for information to get from the eye to the brain (if all is normal); the VEP represents the brain's response to the visual stimulus. The patient is tested many times (maybe 200) and the results are averaged.

58. a) The simplest VEP uses only 3 scalp electrodes. Other methods may involve as many as 12. The eyes are tested separately; the untested eye should be thoroughly occluded so there is no possibility of stimulating it during testing. During flash-VEP, the patient is seated at a Ganzfeld bowl. For the pattern-VEP the patient wears his or her best correction and looks at the monitor screen. Dilation or inadequate correction means that the pattern is not as clear, nor is contrast as good; this results in decreased occipital stimulation.

59. a) If the patient's visual acuity is worse than 20/400 during the recording session, there will be no response on VEP testing. Poor visual acuity may be based on organic pathology such as macular degeneration or uncorrected refractive error. Another possibility is that the patient has not been cooperating and watching the pattern as instructed; poor cooperation may be based on such things as age (the very young and very old may have difficulty fixating on the stimulus for a prolonged period of time) or malingering. (Malingering is the deliberate attempt to fool the examiner.) Some patients who malinger will have undergone VEP testing on numerous occasions, and therefore may be aware of what the pattern VEP is testing for. The flash VEP will always be normal in those who are malingering, but the pattern VEP may be non-recordable based on poor fixation. Individuals with normal vision will have a robust response to both small and large checks. If a patient does not have a response to the very largest check, he or she will be unlikely to have a response to smaller checks. This is not true 100% of the time, but it is extremely rare for a person to have no response to the largest check while having a robust response to smaller checks. If this does occur, it is usually due to poor fixation or fatigue and not to ocular conditions. Finally, a response to the largest check would be expected in all individuals with normal visual acuity, so a non-recordable pattern response would not be considered normal.

60. c) Because the VEP is objective, it can be used where there is a question about whether or not the patient's apparently decreased visual acuity is, in fact, due to a disorder within the visual system. This holds true for both the adult malingerer and the pre-verbal child. (However, since cooperation is a factor in getting a good test, an abnormal result must be considered with care. This is especially true if the pattern response is non-recordable.) It is also used to evaluate

optic nerve disease and visual cortex abnormalities. When combined with information from an ERG and/or EOG, the VEP can help differentiate between retinal problems and problems with the visual pathway. In demyelinating diseases (such as multiple sclerosis), the transmission of the signals will be noticeably slowed. *Note*: As with the flicker-fusion EOG, the flash-VEP may precipitate seizures in patients with epilepsy.

61. d) The flash VEP generates a number of waves (hence the term "complex") each with a positive peak (P) and a negative peak (N) or trough. These waves are distinguished from background brain noise by sheer repetition. The waveform generated by the pattern VEP is a single wave. In both types of VEP testing, the amplitude and latency of the waves are examined.

62. b) The rod photoreceptors are "bleached" by bright light. When a person goes into the dark, it takes a while for the rods to become fully adapted. Dark adaptometry measures the length of time and extent of dark adaptation. The Godmann-Weekers dark adaptometer is usually used; it looks something like a Goldmann perimeter. The time it takes the eye to first note the dim test light is documented. This indicates how long it takes the eye to recover from being light bleached. The test also shows cone adaptation as well. These two features are important, but are not the *primary* reason for performing the test. The *primary* reason is to test how well the rods dark-adapt over time.

63. c) While dark adaptometry is characteristically ordered in the presence (or suspicion) of rod disorders, it also gives information about cone function because the first part of the test measures the dark adaptability of the macula. (See Question 65.) Since this is a subjective test, malingering may be hard to detect. In many instances the malingerer will give inaccurate responses, thus producing a technically unsatisfactory dark adaptometry examination. Other individuals who are not malingering can also produce similar, unsatisfactory results. These include small children, the developmentally delayed, or the very old.

64. c) First, the patient is dark adapted for 2 minutes. Then he or she places the chin in the cup of the adaptometer and is light adapted for 5 minutes. This is done to totally bleach the rods (ie, "burn off" any remaining pigment) and fully stimulate the cones. Full dark adaptation occurs by the end of the dark adapting phase, not at its beginning.

65. a) During the first 5 minutes of dark adaptation, the patient looks straight ahead and is asked to report when he or she first sees a dimly lit target at the back of the bowl. When the patient sees the target, the target is turned off, leaving the patient in darkness again. In 30 seconds (or less) the target is turned on again, and again the patient reports when it is first seen. This is repeated every 30 seconds for about 5 minutes. (This mainly tests the cones because the patient is looking directly at the target with the cone-rich macula.) After 5 minutes, the patient is asked to look at a small red light situated about 2 inches above the target, and again asked to report when the target becomes visible. By shifting the patient's gaze to the red fixation light (which now falls on the macula), the target now falls on the rod-rich peripheral retina.

66. c) Dark adaptometry yields two curves. The first curve, which is short and fast (time is represented on the tracing), represents cone adaptation. The second curve, which is longer and much slower, is the rod adaptation. The point where the two curves cross is known as the rod-cone break. Individuals who have extremely abnormal cones or rods will not produce a rod-cone break. Those with abnormal cones will not show a fast curve initially after the light

has been extinguished. Instead, there will be a slow curve present representing the slowly adapting rods. Individuals with poor rod function will usually show a normal cone curve, but there will be no increase in retinal sensitivity over time (generated by the rods). Thus, there will be no rod curve present on the tracing.

67. d) In disorders where there is no rod function, it is typical for the cone curve to be normal with no rod curve. In these patients, vision in the dark does not improve with time . . . there is no dark adaptation.

68. b) The purpose of the macular photostress test is to determine how quickly the patient's central vision will return to *one acuity line above normal* (for that individual) after a bright light is shown into the eye. The bright light (a transilluminator or direct ophthalmoscope can be used) bleaches the visual pigments from the macular area. One eye is covered, and the light is shown into the fellow eye for 10 seconds. Timing starts once the light is turned off. The measurement reveals the length of time it takes the eye to resynthesize pigment.

69. c) According to Van Boemel, the normal eye will recover to one acuity line above normal in less than 50 seconds. If there is a difference of 20 seconds or more between the patient's eyes, the eye with the longer time is suspicious of having retinal disease. The test can be used to differentiate between macular and optic nerve disease, because optic nerve disorders will still have a normal recovery time.

70. d) The Potential Acuity Meter transmits a tiny, bright eye chart to the back of the eye, bypassing media opacities. Its most common use is in evaluating macular function in the presence of cataracts (especially very dense ones where the physician has a hard time viewing the macula directly).

71. b) There is a knob on the side of the unit where you must dial in the spherical equivalent of the patient's refractive error.

72. b) An infrared light source is used because it will not cause a pupillary response (as would an ordinary flash or room light). Another important feature of the infrared light is that a shadow of the pupil may be seen even if corneal opacities are present. It is worth noting that this test has not been used for a long time. Of the many fine references I used in writing this book, Van Boemel was the only one who mentioned it.

73. b) Since the goal of pupillography is to record pupillary responses, the pupil is not dilated.

74. b) The data obtained on the videotape (or film) is put on a graph, which represents the pupillary response over time (in seconds). The speed of the pupil's reaction is shown on the graph.

75. b) The indirect ophthalmoscope provides a 45 degree field of view. The direct offers only 10 degrees, the Hruby around 20, and the minus contact lens (used with the slit lamp) about 30. Please refer to Table 11-11.

76. c) The green filter is also called a "red-free" filter. When using it, red objects (ie, blood vessels) appear black, increasing their contrast and visibility. The green filter may cause tiny aneurysms to show up, which might be missed when using ordinary light.

77. a) The slit is used to evaluate retinal lesions. The slit is directed so that it falls across the lesion as well as onto normal retina. If the lesion is flat, the line will not be distorted. If the lesion is elevated or depressed, the slit beam will curve.

Table 11-11
Comparison of Direct and Indirect Ophthalmoscopy

Direct	Indirect
Dilated or undilated pupil	Widely dilated pupil
Monocular view	Binocular stereroscopic view
Small field of view (approximately 10 degrees)	Larger 45 degree field of view
Approximately 14X magnification	2X to 4X depending on lens used
Upright, non-reversed view	Inverted and reversed view
Hand-held	Worn on the head of the examiner
No condensing lens necessary	Hand-held condensing lens necessary

(Reprinted with permission from Van Boemel GB. *Special Skills and Techniques*. Thorofare, NJ: SLACK Incorporated; 1999.)

78. b) Scleral depression is used to push structures anterior to the equator down into view. (This area could not be seen without scleral depression and the indirect.)

79. d) The items listed actually refer to the direct ophthalmoscope. See Table 11-11.

80. c) In addition to evaluating the vitreous, macula, optic nerve, and retinal vessels, the fundus exam also gives information on media clarity. The color and brightness (and presence or absence) of the fundus reflex can be diagnostic. And, of course, the optic nerve is evaluated for a cup-to-disc ratio.

81. a) The optical section of the light source is what makes the slit lamp so unique, and what specifically qualifies it for examination of the eye. The other items are nice, but without the optical section, examination of the eye (and especially of the cornea) would not be what it is today.

82. d) At 40X, it will be difficult to orient yourself at first. In addition, even very tiny movements on the patient's part will be greatly magnified, causing the eye to "swoosh" in front of you. Start with a lower power. This will enable you to focus the instrument quickly and to locate the areas of specific interest. Once that is done, then you can increase the magnification. Please refer to Table 11-12 for more examination information.

83. c) Puzzled? Answers b and d are diagnoses, not findings. Answer a is an abbreviation that lawyers laugh at and say that it means "we never looked," although it is supposed to mean "within normal limits." While you might be able to squeak by with Answer a, Answer c is the best because it simply describes what is seen and does not make a diagnosis. (Remember, diagnosing is outside the legal realm of ophthalmic medical personnel at any certification level.)

84. b) A direct, narrow beam (the narrowest available) directed at the limbus from about 60 degrees is used to evaluate chamber depth. This method puts a sharply focused beam of light on the cornea and an unfocused beam on the iris. The dark band in between these two is the object of your interest, because it represents the depth of the anterior chamber (ie, the space between the cornea and iris). Compare the width of the shadow to the width of the corneal band. If the shadow is one fourth to one half as wide as the corneal band, then the angle is

---

Table 11-12
Slit Lamp Examination

Suggested Power

6X or 10X	external (lids, conjunctiva), contact lenses
16X	angles, cornea, lens, foreign bodies, corneal abrasions
40X	corneal endothelium

Beam Width

1 Narrowest	angles, cornea, anterior chamber
2 A bit wider	cornea, lens, etc
3 A bit wider yet	external, contact lenses
4 Full width	external, applanation tension (with blue filter)

Beam Height

Full	most areas and structures
Short	checking anterior chamber for cells and flare

Color/Filter

White	most areas and structures
Blue	(use fluorescein dye) applanation tensions, corneal staining, tear film, staining patterns of rigid contact lenses
Green (red-free)	evaluating blood vessels, iron lines
Diffuser	general viewing of the eye as a whole, orientation
Wratten filter	contact lens evaluation (along with blue filter)

(Modified from Ledford JK, Sanders V. *The Slit Lamp Primer*. Thorofare, NJ: SLACK Incorporated; 1998.)

---

open (or the chamber is deep). If the shadow is less than one fourth that of the corneal band, then the angle is narrow (or the chamber is shallow). If the shadow is missing, then the cornea and iris are so close together that the angle is closed or nearly closed (or the chamber is flat). *Note*: For more on slit lamp illumination techniques, see Table 11-7.

85. c) The Wratten filter is also called a #12 yellow filter. It enhances the color of the fluorescein by blocking out excess blue light. (By the way, the green filter *is* red-free. It is used when viewing blood vessels, among other things. See Table 11-12.)

86. d) The Hruby lens is a slit lamp attachment that can be used to view a limited portion of the posterior pole (eg, for cup-to-disc ratios). A contact fundus lens can also be used.

87. b) Like Placido's disk, the photokeratoscope utilizes a pattern of concentric rings which are projected onto the anterior surface of the cornea. As the name implies, photographs of the reflection can be made for documentation. Its uses include the evaluation of postoperative astigmatism and keratoconus.

88. b) The patient should be told to blink just prior to the picture being taken in order to moisten the corneal surface. A dry cornea can cause false irregularities (artifacts) to appear on the photo.

89. a) Alignment and proper focus are the keys in performing quality photokeratoscopy. The central cornea must be centered and sharply focused, otherwise the results are inaccurate.

90. c) This is easier to understand if you think of a topographical map. If one looks at such a map of a steep mountain, the lines are close together. If the map shows a gently rolling hill, the lines will be spaced farther apart.

91. a) This photograph is of a patient who has keratoconus. The inferior cornea is steeper as noted by the narrowness of the space between rings.

92. b) Pachymetry is usually performed with an ultrasonic measurement. There is an optical pachymeter which uses the slit lamp, but in general the ultrasonic instrument is easier to use and more portable.

93. d) The probe must be held perpendicular to the portion of the corneal surface being measured. When measuring central cornea, this is not too difficult. The hard part is measuring the periphery, where the cornea is more curved.

94. c) The thickness of the cornea is vital information in refractive surgery, where instruments are used to alter the shape of the cornea in order to change the patient's refractive error. An error could result in a perforation or inaccurate correction.

95. b) The central cornea should be the easiest to measure, since it is easier to maintain proper alignment in this position. It is also the thinnest part of the cornea, providing a number with which to compare subsequent readings. Therefore it is best to start the measurements with the central cornea.

96. d) The charts for *near* testing of low vision provide continuous text, not the distance charts. The "normal" Snellen distance charts usually jump from 20/100 to 20/200 to 20/400. A distant chart for low vision patients provides several rows of letters (or test objects) that fall between these gradations.
    Note: This is one of the more ambiguous entries in the Criteria. Refractometry of low vision patients and low vision aids are covered in Chapter 5. Definitions of sub-normal vision categories are found in Chapter 10. It is somewhat unclear what JCAHPO means by "Low Vision Equipment." It might be worth noting that if you are setting up a low vision clinic, you will need a set of magnifiers (hand-held, head-born, and other), a stock of non-optical devices (large print items, needle threaders, etc), reading stands, and lamps . . . perhaps these are what qualify as "equipment."

97. a) When testing near acuity in the low vision patient, we are more concerned with functional ability. For this reason, a card with continuous text is used instead of one with rows of isolated letters.

98. d) The contrast sensitivity test is used in some cases to help determine the magnification of low vision aids. The results of the glare test might indicate a need for tinted lenses. Amsler grid testing is used to map out any central scotomata and also to note any areas of distortion.

99. c) The standard Snellen chart employs black letters on a bright, white background. In other words, it has high contrast. How much of our world is of such high contrast? Most of what we look at are shades and shadows. Therefore, the Snellen chart may give an exaggerated sense of the patient's acuity. Low contrast situations which are difficult for a person with normal contrast sensitivity may be virtually debilitating to a person with low contrast sensitivity.

100. a) Various test objects have been used as targets for contrast sensitivity testing, including letters (including tumbling E's), objects, and gratings. The objects generally go gradually from high-contrast to low-contrast on a graduated scale. The patient is requested to identify the faintest object (ie, the one with the lowest contrast) possible. When gratings are used, not only is the contrast graduated, but the lines in the gratings are varied from wide to moderate to narrow. This gives more detailed information.

101. c) The patient should be provided with best correction. If the "best" correction is his or her glasses, then the habitual correction may be worn . . . *provided that the lenses are not tinted* (which may reduce the patient's ability to discern subtle contrasts). If the glasses are tinted and/or do not provide the best acuity, then use a trial frame.

102. a) The patient should be urged to guess when nearing his or her contrast threshold. If the patient is allowed to respond only when sure of the answers, the measurement will be artificially decreased. You must judge the patient's threshold by noting the point at which "guessed-at" answers begin to be consistently wrong.

103. b) The contrast of the gratings vary and are assigned percentages (eg, 50% contrast or 30% contrast). The width of the bands also varies, based on cycles per degree (c/d). (This is also called spatial frequencies.) The higher the frequency of grating, the more bars in the circle. Generally, the frequency gets higher as you go down the chart. The contrast goes down as you go from left to right. This has all been developed scientifically. Once the test is done, the information is used to plot the patient's contrast sensitivity curve. Van Boemel notes that score sheets from one type of test may not be accurate when used with another type of test.

104. c) At this point you will not see physicians making definitive diagnoses on the basis of contrast sensitivity testing alone because the frequency losses caused by various disorders tends to overlap. However, according to Van Boemel, some implications can be made. She states that sensitivity loss in the higher frequencies are often associated with macular, corneal, and lenticular problems. Losses in the mid-range are often associated with optic nerve disorders. Finally, a decrease in the lower frequencies are often related to disorders involving the brain. A study of my reference material seems to show that there are disagreements among the professionals regarding the usefulness of contrast sensitivity testing beyond showing a need for cataract surgery (when Snellen acuities do not seem to indicate that need).

Chapter 10. Advanced General Medical Knowledge

1. b) Diabetes causes tiny areas of bulging in the retinal blood vessels. These bulges are known as aneurysms (termed "micro" because they are so small). Aneurysms tend to leak fluid and sometimes burst, causing hemorrhages.

2. b) When fluid leaks from microaneurysms and other diabetes-weakened retinal vessels, retinal swelling occurs. If the macula is involved, vision will be affected. Bittinger states that macular edema is the leading cause of blindness in diabetics.

3. a) The body forms new blood vessels (neo = new, vascularization refers to the vascular system) in an attempt to get blood flow (and oxygen) to the tissues. Unfortunately, the new blood vessels are faulty and weak, prone to leakage and rupture.

4. d) Background diabetic retinopathy involves microaneurysms (see Question 1), hemorrhages, cotton-wool spots (areas of tissue death), and hard exudates (fluid that has leaked out of the vessels). Proliferative retinopathy involves these plus the appearance of neovascularization and hemorrhages from the retinal veins (including vitreous hemorrhages). (By the way, any time you see the word *only* [or *always* or *never*] in an answer, that answer is almost guaranteed to be incorrect!)

5. c) Pavan-Langston states that the main factor in the occurrence of retinopathy related to diabetes is the duration of the diabetes. She states that "two-thirds of those with diabetes for 15 years or more . . ." have retinopathy. While not mentioned here, the level of sugar control maintained by the patient has long been touted by physicians as a key in preventing or retarding retinopathy, but this issue is not proven, nor do the experts agree. However, Pavan-Langston notes that "it is generally assumed that good control delays the onset of retinopathy."

6. c) Cataracts occur earlier and more often in diabetics. Changes in the patient's refractometric measurement occur in cases where the blood sugar level is not well controlled. In theory, diabetes works like this. First, the patient's blood sugar becomes elevated. In an effort to try to equalize the sugar content of the body tissues, water is taken out of the tissues and added to the bloodstream. (One sign of diabetes is frequent urination, a result of this added fluid.) The lens of the eye is not exempt from this tissue dehydration. This dehydration of the lens causes an increase in the curvature of the lens surfaces, which is responsible for the shift toward myopia. Finally, nerve palsies can occur. The third, fourth, and sixth nerves may be affected; the patient complains of diplopia.

7. a) In the first stages of hypertensive retinopathy, the walls of the retinal blood vessels become fibrous. This changes the way that the vessels reflect light, causing them to look silver- or copper-lined (hence the common terms "copper" or "silver" wiring). It is worth mentioning that hypertensive retinopathy has been divided into four stages known as the Keith-Wagener-Barker classification system. Group I exhibits copper or silver wiring. Group II demonstrates AV crossing (see Question 8) and sometimes hard exudates and tiny hemorrhages. Group III exhibits retinal edema, hemorrhages, and cotton-wool spots. Group IV has the problems of Group III with the addition of disk edema.

8. b) In later stages of hypertensive retinopathy, the retinal vessels may be straightened or twisted (often referred to as *tortuous*). Overlying arteries may push into the veins where they cross over ("AV crossing"), causing a narrowing of the veins in that area ("AV nicking").

9. c) Pavan-Langston notes that serious loss of vision "does not usually occur as a direct result of the hypertensive process unless there is local arterial or venous occlusion."

10. c) Vaughan, Asbury, and Riordan-Eva state that "resolution of the cotton-wool spots and the arteriolar changes occurs with successful hypotensive therapy."

11. a) In atherosclerosis, fat builds up in the arteries, which can include the arteries of the eye. This fatty build-up is called an atheroma. Either the atheroma builds up to the point of obstructing the artery, or a piece of fatty plaque (from anywhere in the body) breaks free, travels to the eye, and becomes lodged in an artery, blocking it off. (It might be worth noting that the term *atherosclerosis* refers to this fatty build-up in larger arteries [larger than 300 microns]. In smaller vessels [including the retinal arterioles, which are less than 30 microns], the disorder is

called *arteriosclerosis*. The central retinal artery is large enough to be involved in atherosclerosis. In addition, arteriolosclerosis is characteristically associated with hypertension, while atherosclerosis is not.)

12. c) Pavan-Langston makes this statement. She adds that the most common cause in children is "probably" orbital cellulitis vs neoplasm.

13. b) In Graves' disease (associated with hyperthyroidism), the extraocular muscles become inflamed and swollen. This swelling forces the eyeball outward, causing exophthalmus. Exophthalmus may progress to the point where the upper lid can no longer close over the globe, creating problems with exposure.

14. a) These signs are related to the inflammation of extraocular muscles as discussed in Question 13.

15. d) The items in the answer probably sound like an odd combination. Corneal dryness (with possible subsequent abrasions, ulcers, etc) is caused by lack of lid closure (see Question 13). Optic nerve compression is caused by the swollen extraocular muscles.

16. d) The inflamed muscles may become fibrotic and begin to atrophy. Limitations on upgaze are often caused by adhesions between the IR and IO muscles. The swelling of the inflamed EOMs may also restrict movement. Vaughan, Asbury, and Riordan-Eva note that if the patient's IOP is lower in primary gaze than it is in upgaze, then an adhesion may, indeed, exist.

17. a) The answer seems rather bizarre, but true (these are listed by Bittinger). Pavan-Langston also lists photophobia, periorbital edema, eyelid edema, and optic neuritis. A more common finding, however, is a loss of the outer one third of the eyebrows.

18. c) Because the pituitary gland is located right below the optic chiasm, the growth of a pituitary tumor (also called a pituitary adenoma) may put pressure on the chiasm, causing visual field defects.

19. c) The nasal fibers from both retinas cross in the chiasm. Since the nasal fibers are responsible for the temporal field, pressure in this area causes a disturbance in the temporal fields (generally of both eyes).

20. a) If the pressure on the chiasm is relieved at an early stage, the visual field loss generally reverses. However, continued pressure can cause atrophy of the optic nerve with associated permanent vision loss.

21. b) Cushing's syndrome is caused by high levels of pituitary hormones. Ocular manifestations of Cushing's can include exophthalmus, papilledema, and retinal hemorrhages and exudates. Some of these problems area caused by associated hypertension. (The list comes from Pavan-Langston.)

22. a) Because the brain is encased in the skull with little room for expansion, many of the symptoms caused by brain tumors are due to an elevation in the pressure inside the head.

23. d) These symptoms do not assist the physician in locating a brain lesion because they are actually symptoms of increased intracranial pressure caused by the tumor. (Did you notice that the items in Answer c were signs, not symptoms? Reading a question carefully can help you rule out certain answers.)

24. c) Areas for ocular pursuit movements are located in the occipital lobe, thus abnormal optokinetic ability and nystagmus may be present.

25. a) Amaurosis fugax is a temporary, painless loss of vision in one eye caused by obstruction of retinal blood vessels. The obstruction is generally caused by an embolus (cholesterol, calcific, or platelets). Disorders often associated with amaurosis fugax are carotid artery disease, atherosclerosis, heart valve damage, endocarditis, anemia, and sickle cell disease. (This list is from Vaughan, Asbury, and Riordan-Eva.)

26. b) Herpes zoster virus (also called shingles) occurs in people with a history of previous infection with chicken pox (varicella-zoster). Shingles occur on one side and are often quite painful. Episcleritis and uveitis may also occur with the infection. If there is a lesion on the tip of the nose, corneal involvement is certain. While Answer d is possible, contact dermatitis is not necessarily painful, nor does it respect the midline of the face.

27. c) According to Vaughan, Asbury, and Riordan-Eva, the most common ocular findings in AIDS are changes in the retinal blood vessels (with hemorrhages and cotton-wool spots) and changes in the conjunctival blood vessels (the appearance of tiny, curved vessels as well as linear hemorrhages). They also report that while the primary systemic problem in AIDS is frequent infections, the eye is involved in these infections in only about 30% of cases.

28. d) Sjogren's syndrome is most often associated with rheumatoid arthritis, and includes severe dry eye as well as dry mouth. Other ocular manifestations associated with rheumatoid arthritis are scleritis and episcleritis. Medications used to treat rheumatoid arthritis (such as steroids) can also cause ocular problems.

29. a) According to Bittinger, lack of vitamin A is what causes the most severe ocular problems in malnutrition. Vitamin A deficiency in the eye can cause xerophthalmia, a catch-all phrase that includes night blindness, retinopathy, and ulceration of the cornea. In its final stages, xerophthalmia progresses to keratomalacia, where the corneal tissue dies.

30. d) While smoking has the effects listed in every answer, the most common problem is chronic irritation caused by exposure to smoke (Bittinger).

31. b) The elevated IOP seen in gout may well be associated with the use of steroids by those with the disorder. Ocular injection seen in patients with gout may be related to scleritis, episcleritis, or conjunctivitis.

32. a) You might suspect this answer, since multiple sclerosis is a nerve disorder. During acute optic neuritis, the patient may have blurred vision and/or a central scotoma. If the nerves to the EOMs become involved, the patient may experience diplopia or nystagmus. Ptosis can also occur.

33. b) Myasthenia gravis affects the striated muscles (generally, those involved in movement), which fatigue easily. If the EOMs are affected, diplopia results. If the levator is affected, ptosis occurs. (Ptosis that is caused by myasthenia can be detected by a Tensilon [ICN Pharmaceuticals, Costa Mesa, Calif] test, see Chapter 8, Question 41.) Abnormal pupil size may also occur.

34. c) The patient with Marfan's syndrome is generally lean and tall, with long fingers and toes. The eye is often involved, particularly dislocation of the lens.

35. a) The use of systemic steroids for various inflammatory disorders can be the cause of secondary glaucoma.

36. c) Legal blindness is defined as having vision of 20/200 (or worse) as the best corrected vision in the best eye. (This is with traditional correction, without the use of any low vision aids.) It also exists if the patient's visual field is restricted to 20 degrees or less. Remember, "low vision" is not defined by laws and regulations; "legal blindness" is. Also remember that "legal blindness" includes both the partially sighted and the totally blind.

37. c) While being legally blind is necessary to receive free government assistance, the federal registry still recognizes the fact that, while a person may not be legally blind, he may still be disabled. Such a person may qualify for some type of insurance, social services, or Social Security compensation.

38. d) When using tables to figure the degree of a patient's visual disability, in addition to distant and near acuity and visual fields, one may figure in an extra percentage if the patient is aphakic or pseudophakic in one eye. Restricted range of motion and diplopia can also be figured in. (Appendix A in Van Boemel's book describes how to figure visual disability.)

39. d) Unfortunately, many causes of legal blindness are age related. More elderly adults fall into the category of legal blindness than the other groups listed. (Stein, Slatt, and Stein note that 70% of the legally and totally blind are age 65 and older.)

40. c) Retinal disorders (including diabetic retinopathy and macular degeneration) are the leading cause of blindness in adults in the Western world according to Foster. He also notes that the leading causes of blindness in children are also retinal, but of a different sort, due to inherited ocular disorders and prematurity.

41. d) Cortical blindness (also called cerebral blindness) occurs in the visual pathway at some point beyond the geniculate body. Thus the patient has normal pupils, clear media, and a normal-appearing fundus. It can be associated with stroke, multiple sclerosis, meningitis, encephalitis, electrical injury, mercury or lead poisoning, head trauma, brain tumor, or other problems. (This information came from Lessell, Lessell, and Glaser.)

42. a) Stein, Slatt, and Stein report that of the legally blind persons in the United States and Canada, about 75% of them have some residual vision. The other 25% are totally blind (ie, have no light perception).

43. c) Obviously, someone who is totally blind will need to use non-optical aids (talking watch, Braille, etc). Mobility training is also important to help the patient ambulate confidently. Some type of counseling may be needed to help the patient cope with his or her visual loss (or life in general). Vocational rehabilitation (although not part of a correct answer) may also be required to assist the patient in adapting to a new job. Contact with the appropriate social services is also important. Annual eye exams are important, but are not a part of rehabilitation.

44. d) Each of these items contributes to the usefulness of the legally blind patient's remaining vision. (See also Chapter 9, Question 98.)

45. c) The low vision patient is not encouraged to guess at the letters because we are concerned with functional vision. (Reviewer Brown notes, however, that guessing is useful in order to

know the patient's visual threshold . . . so opinions vary.) Use a near card of continuous text rather than single letters or numbers. The acuity to record is the last line that the patient can read with ease.

46. a) Visual efficiency can actually be calculated from the patient's central acuity and peripheral field using tables and a simple formula. Ocular motility (but not stereopsis) is also sometimes figured in. For the curious, the method is detailed in Van Boemel's book.

47. c) Vision is a major part of our lives. Loosing it (whether suddenly or gradually) will naturally involve a grieving process, which might include denial, hostility, anxiety, fear, and sadness. The patient (and family) should be reassured that these reactions are normal. The patient will usually have to work through the grief before being ready for rehabilitation.

48. b) Some patients have the mistaken idea that they have caused their poor vision by overusing their eyes. Also, one of the biggest fears of low vision patients is that they will go totally blind. Although you cannot always convince them, they should be reassured that they did not cause the problem, and that using their eyes will not cause more damage.

49. c) This question was about misconceptions. First, it is a common myth that the other senses of a blind person will become more acute. This is not true. What is true is that the patient must learn to rely more on the other senses; the problem here is that we usually use our vision to validate input from the other senses (you hear a noise and turn to see what made it). It is a challenge for the visually disabled to find new ways to be useful and independent; this is not easy . . . but it certainly is possible. And even those who love them best may now find it hard to include them; the visually impaired may be totally excluded from an activity, the attitudes of others may now include pity, or they are treated differently (eg, people talk louder). What is true is that the visually impaired may have to find new recreational outlets for relaxation and stress relief. While perhaps difficult, this is not impossible. Adjusting takes time.

50. c) The best way to find out what the low vision patient needs is to ask him or her, which is part of the history-taking process. You might ask the patient, "What one thing would you like to be able to do that you can't do now?" He or she may suggest an activity that is not possible (even with low vision aids), but if you keep asking, you will eventually find a need you can help meet. Regardless of how careful your measurements and observations, if a low vision aid does not meet the patient's perception of his or her own needs, it will not be accepted. (Brown's book offers excellent information on this topic.)

51. c) Repetitive activities such as rocking, waving the hands, and rubbing the eyes are known as blindisms. Pushing on the eyes may stimulate the retinas, giving visual sensations of light.

52. c) Trachoma is not difficult to treat . . . all it requires is sulfonamides or tetracycline drugs.

53. a) According to Pavan-Langston, toxoplasmosis "is the most common proved cause of chorioretinitis in the world." It is usually congenital, but in rare cases may be acquired. The disorder is caused by *Toxoplasma gondii*. The oocyst may be present in cat feces, but it may also be airborne or present in the soil or in undercooked meat. The organism can affect the whole central nervous system or be confined to the eye. In the eye, retinal cysts form. These may scar the retina or become active and cause chorioretinitis.

54. d) Generally, the patient with EKC does not have any systemic symptoms. As its name implies, EKC is highly contagious. The conjunctivitis itself lasts from 1 to 2 weeks. The keratitis involves epithelial defects that stain and subsequently turn opaque.

55. c) Orbital cellulitis usually occurs as infection spreads from the ethmoid sinuses. The most common organisms involved are *Staphylococcus*, *Streptococcus*, and *Haemophilus*. Signs and symptoms include swelling, pain, tenderness, and fever. There may be some restriction of eye movements. When exophthalmus is seen in a child, orbital cellulitis is the most common cause. In severe cases, the infection can erode the orbital bones and cause brain abscesses and meningitis. Thus prompt treatment is necessary.

56. c) Sympathetic ophthalmia occurs in the non-insulted eye following trauma (or sometimes surgery) of the other eye. It is a bilateral uveitis, and may occur 10 days to years after the original injury. (Most cases, however, occur within 1 year.) Blindness in both eyes can occur in months (or sometimes years) if the disorder is allowed to progress untreated. Once the scenario has begun, enucleating the insulted eye will not stop the disorder's progression in the fellow eye; this is why a severely damaged eye is enucleated within 10 days of the injury.

57. a) While endophthalmitis can occur following trauma, most cases occur postoperatively. This is usually due to bacteria (most notably *Staphylococcus aureus*), but may also be caused by fungi. There is a form of sterile endophthalmitis that is due to retained foreign bodies (such as powder from surgical gloves), irritating chemicals, or manipulation of the vitreous.

58. c) Corneal infiltrates are an accumulation of fluid and inflammatory cells just below the epithelial surface, thus they do not stain. A sterile infiltrate, seen sometimes in contact lens wearers, can be an allergic or chemical reaction (as to contact lens solutions).

59. a) Vernal conjunctivitis *is* seasonal, but it occurs during the warm months, not the cold ones.

60. a) A coloboma occurs when structures fail to fuse during embryologic development. Involved structures may include the lid, the iris, the choroid, the optic nerve, and/or the retina.

61. c) Retinopathy of prematurity is mainly due to oxygen toxicity. The retinal vessels form from the optic disk outward starting during the fourth month of gestation and continuing through months eight and nine. When oxygen is given in excess before the process is complete, the newly forming vessels are obliterated.

62. d) The word "always" in Answer d should have given this away, as well as the information in Answer a. There are two types of albinism. The type that involves the skin and eye (oculocutaneous) does have pink skin and white hair. Those with ocular albinism have normal skin and hair pigment, but pigmentation in the eye is deficient. Thus they have light irides and the macula is underdeveloped. In addition, ocular albinism is X-linked recessive, so females carry it without symptoms, but the males who inherit the genes exhibit the symptoms.

63. a) The capillary hemangioma (also called a strawberry nevus) is the most common congenital vascular tumor. These appear at birth or shortly thereafter, tend to grow rapidly, then disappear around age 7. No treatment is recommended unless the tumor is causing pupillary obstruction. A port wine stain is a type of hemangioma, but is not a capillary hemangioma; it does not grow or regress.

64. d) The papilloma is an area of thickened epithelium. They are sometimes pigmented, but they are the most common of the benign lid tumors.

65. b) A malignant melanoma may occur on the lids or conjunctiva, arising from a nevus or occurring spontaneously. The intraocular melanoma, however, occurs only in the uveal tract. It may cause forward displacement of the lens and precipitate angle closure. Uveal melanoma can also cause secondary glaucoma by pigment dispersion blocking the angle or by stimulating neovascularization in the angle. Pavan-Langston says that the malignant melanoma is the most common intraocular tumor seen in adults (usually appearing after age 50).

66. d) Whether a nevus is flat or raised is not a danger signal. You should look for ABCD:
A—asymmetry; one half of the lesion does not match the other half
B—border; the lesion's borders are jagged, blurred, or irregular
C—color; more than one color is present (shades of tan, brown, and black, or flecks of white, red, or blue)
D—diameter; keep an eye on any lesion larger than 0.25 inch
In addition, skin cancers may have a center dimple, pearly edges, and/or crusting and bleeding.

67. c) Retinoblastoma is a congenital (and genetic) malignant tumor of the photoreceptor cells. It is often undiagnosed in its early stages; however, it is usually found by age 3. Leukocoria ("white pupil") and strabismus are often the presenting symptoms. (However, Vaughan, Asbury, and Riordan-Eva note that congenital cataracts and retinopathy of prematurity cause most cases of leukocoria.)

68. d) Fuch's epithelial-endothelial dystrophy generally occurs in women starting in their 30s and 40s. Decompensation of the endothelium leads to stromal edema, causing decreased vision. Topical hypertonic sodium chloride is used to try to decrease the edema. If edema progresses to the epithelium, painful bullous keratopathy can result. (*Note*: Fingerprint and map-dot dystrophies occur in Bowman's membrane, and generally have no visual symptoms. Ectatic dystrophy is another name for keratoconus.)

69. b) According to Vaughan, Asbury, and Riordan-Eva, intraocular surgery is the entity most often associated with cystoid macular edema. It is usually evident within the 4th to 12th postoperative week, but may occur months or years later. Any postoperative patient who experiences a decrease in vision should be suspected of developing cystoid macular edema. However, Wilson and Wilson note that postoperative patients may exhibit cystoid macular edema on fundoscopy yet experience no vision decrease. The disorder is best displayed with fluorescein angiography, where a rosette or flower petal pattern appears around the macula.

70. b) Syneresis is the shrinking of the vitreous gel, usually associated with age (60 years and over) but sometimes occurring in childhood, especially in myopes. It may *cause* posterior vitreous detachment and/or vitreous collapse. (*Note*: Asteroid hyalosis is the presence of calcium soap particles in the vitreous. They are highly reflective, showing up nicely on slit lamp examination, but have little if any affect on the patient's vision.)

71. b) Seidel's test is done while observing through the slit lamp. It involves touching a moistened fluorescein strip directly to the area in question. If there is leaking aqueous, it will dilute the fluorescein, producing a thin stream of green where the aqueous is flowing out.

72. c) A concussion type of injury is caused by the force of a blow as that force is conducted through the tissues. This type of injury might be seen in a motor vehicle accident or an explosion, and is not caused by direct contact but rather by the waves of the force traveling through the body. (A contusion is caused by direct contact.)

73. b) Vossius' ring is a ring of pigment that is imprinted onto the anterior lens capsule surface when the iris is forced back onto the lens during a concussive injury. The pigment may disperse with time.

74. d) Siderosis is the condition caused by a retained iron intraocular foreign body. Pavan-Langston notes that "Retained iron . . . undergoes electrolytic decomposition, combines with tissue cells, and causes eventual cell death." This can be especially devastating to the retina. In later stages, as with this patient, one might see heterochromia, cataract, and secondary glaucoma. Also from Pavan-Langston is this list that you may find useful:
    Metallic Foreign Bodies
    Toxic: lead, zinc, nickel, aluminum, copper, iron
    Nontoxic: gold, silver, platinum, tantalum
    Nonmetallic Foreign Bodies
    Toxic: vegetable matter, cloth particles, cilia, eyelid particle
    Nontoxic: stone, glass, porcelain, carbon, some plastics

75. a) The findings given suggest a perforated globe. The brown exudate is prolapsed choroid; the pupil is drawn toward the prolapse, thus its D shape. In addition to decreased vision, other findings in a globe perforation could include hypotony, flat or shallow anterior chamber, marked chemosis, and an obvious laceration in the sclera or cornea.

76. d) A laceration in the lower nasal canthus area most likely involves the punctum and canalicula. If the tissues are not properly approximated and sutured, the tear drainage system could be permanently damaged. The patient would then experience chronic epiphora.

77. c) Enophthalmus is an abnormal backward regression ("retrodisplacement") of the eyeball.

78. b) In angle-recession glaucoma, an episode of blunt trauma has forced a tear in the ciliary muscle, causing the insertion point of the iris to recede. Secondary glaucoma may develop within 8 weeks or up to 15 years later. The elevated IOP is thought to be due to damage to the trabeculum, although the trabeculum may look normal. Initially, angle recession is usually accompanied by a hyphema.

79. a) Commotio retinae (also called Berlin's edema) is retinal swelling that occurs after a blunt or concussive injury to the eye. The swelling occurs on the side opposite the area of impact, thus the visual field loss occurs on the same side as impact. There is no treatment, and vision generally improves slowly over a period of weeks.

Taking a Practical Exam

I can just about guarantee that your practical exam won't be as harrowing as mine. I took my practical back in the days when it was given during the American Academy of Ophthalmology annual meeting. The year I took the exam, the meeting was in Las Vegas. Even though it was a practical, I was still studying written notes in preparation. I had the most essential notes with me on the plane; the rest I packed in my luggage to go over in my motel room that night. (The test was scheduled for the day after I arrived.) I was dressed casually for the trip in blue jeans, tennis shoes, and a pull-over sweater. Several friends from the office were with me, and they were very tolerant of both my studying and my nerves!

We had to change planes in Texas. When we got to Las Vegas, we were tired . . . Nevada is 3 hours behind Georgia. We went to get our luggage only to find out that it had taken the term "jet lag" too seriously . . . it had lagged behind on a jet in Texas.

So much for my other study notes. So much for eye shadow and deodorant. So much for clean clothes.

The next morning I took a taxi to the test site. On the way, I had the cabby stop so I could buy a few essentials. I was still wearing my jeans and tennis shoes . . . not at all the way I'd planned to appear. (You know, first impressions and all that?) But those are the kind of clothes I feel most comfortable in, so I decided it was a bonus. Besides, I couldn't do a thing about it. I was pretty relaxed that day, and a few weeks later I got that treasured note in the mail saying . . . I'd passed! (Moral of the story: pack a carry-on bag with your notes and a change of clothes!)

Surely your experience with the performance exam will go more smoothly than that! So take heart. In this brief section I'm going to share a few tidbits that should help you prepare.

You should obviously practice each of the required skills ahead of time. Be sure to review the performance areas listed in the most current *Certified Ophthalmic Medical Technologist* booklet. Offices vary, and it is likely that some of the items in the performance areas are not tests that are routinely done in your office. It is true that you will not be required to perform every task at the practical, but you have no way of knowing which tasks you'll need to do. Thus, you must be proficient at all of them. (In fact, when you signed up to take the written exam, your ophthalmologist/sponsor signed stating that you were already proficient.)

Several months before the practical, make yourself a notebook and write one skill at the top of each page. Make columns for date, patient name/number (optional), test results, and notes. For example, you may be asked to derive the prescription of a lens using the Geneva lens measure. On that page, you would note the reading you got using the lens clock, then the reading you got using a lensometer to check your work. Under the notes column, make comments about steps you might have forgotten or other adjustments you need to make. (For example, when I kept such a notebook I found that my retinoscopy working lens should be a +1.25 instead of the usual +1.50. I never realized that until I kept a record of my results.)

If your office does not have the equipment to do certain tasks or does not require certain tasks, you will need to be creative. You might see if you can borrow an item from another office or clinic. (For example, there is probably a Tangent screen gathering dust in a closet in some office in town.) If your office isn't into opticianry-type tasks, check with the optician to whom you refer your patients. He or she will be glad to have you come in and use the lens clock and/or show you how to measure a pair of frames. In cases where your practice simply does not do a certain test routinely, discuss the situation with your employer or clinical supervisor. It only takes a few seconds to measure vertex distance. If you measured a couple patients a day for a few weeks, you'd be proficient by the time you took your exam. The key is to find a way to accomplish your goal. Wouldn't it be sad to never become certified only because your office doesn't have a Goldmann perimeter? Find a way around any and all obstacles!

I mentioned earlier that I was still studying written notes in preparation for the exam. This is a good idea. You may still be called upon to identify things in photographs, for example, and studying is appropriate. In addition, you may be performing some tests that you don't usually do in your clinic or that might not be on your job description, so study notes are needed to help you memorize the necessary steps.

Each year JCAHPO makes up a list of the equipment available at the test site. This includes such information as the brand of the instrument. This is helpful because there might be subtle (or not so subtle) differences between, say, a Marco and a B&L brand of the same piece of equipment. If the list shows a different brand than you are familiar with, call around and see if another office has what you need. At least you could spare a few minutes to go look at it. Perhaps you'll simply be reassuring yourself that both instruments are the same. In some cases, if the test site instrumentation is different from yours, you might want to take your own with you. (For example, the test site uses minus cylinder phoropters and you are used to plus. You should know how to use both, of course, but for the exam you will be more relaxed if using something familiar.) If, by chance, the list is not in your information packet from JCAHPO, call or e-mail them and request it.

The preparation steps above need to be started months before the practical. What about test day? There are still things you can do to help yourself. First, if possible, visit the test site. If there's any way, go into the clinic and see the rooms. Being familiar with the rooms will help relieve stress. If that is not possible, at least drive by the office. This will alleviate anxiety about getting lost on test day.

Get a good night's sleep the night before, and get up early enough in the morning to allow yourself plenty of time to get ready. Eat a good breakfast that includes some protein (but don't over-eat!). Wear clothing that is comfortable but professional. While pass/fail is in no way dependent on your attire (and I'm a case in point), it is probably a good idea to dress as if you are going to a job interview. (As a good friend of mine says, "You never know when or where you're going to meet your next boss!" Another friend reminds us that if you are dressed sloppily, it seems to say something about how you regard yourself and your profession.) If there is time and you feel it is necessary, you might glance at your notes one more time.

Remember to take any papers required (including photo ID and your admission pass, if one is issued) and any equipment you have brought with you. Arrive a little early, especially if you did not get to go into the building the day before. Sign in, look around, and breathe deeply.

You'll probably be given a schedule to follow. When moving from one place to another, don't hesitate to ask if you are headed in the right direction. When you arrive in the room, you may introduce yourself to the proctor(s) and patient(s). As someone who has been a skill evaluator myself, I can tell you that these people are on your side. They believe in certification so much that they are willing to get involved. They want you to pass, so don't view them as the enemy!

As much as possible, act as if you are in your own clinic during a normal workday. You would never walk into an exam room and tell the patient, "I've never done this before..." Don't say this to the proctors, either, even if it's true (and it shouldn't be). Nor should you make comments such as, "We use automated lensometers in our office..." or "No one does Goldmann fields any more. I don't see why it's on the test." While such comments won't fail you (you are graded on performance, not attitude), they are not very professional. Keep them to yourself. If you feel that something was truly unfair, and you don't agree with the outcome, you have the right to appeal the situation to JCAHPO. The appeals process is outlined in the criteria booklet.

In cases where you have a list of tasks, if you are allowed to choose your order of performance it is usually best to start with those items with which you are most comfortable. It is also a good idea to first do those tasks that take the least time. This will boost your confidence and reduce the sensation of being rushed. You may ask the proctors questions, although they are very limited as to what they can tell you. But if you are faced with an unfamiliar piece of equipment (which shouldn't happen if you've done your homework), they can tell you where the "on" button is.

Feel free to talk yourself through any task, even aloud. The proctors don't care, and neither does the patient. For example, suppose you are performing retinoscopy. You might say to yourself, "Both apertures are opened. I'm going to dial in the retinoscopy lens. Checking the reflexes. This one has with motion and is bright, wide, and fast . . . add plus sphere. That's neutral. Turn streak 90 degrees . . . this reflex shows with motion. Adjust axis, add plus cylinder . . ." You get the idea.

It is important that you treat the "patient" like a patient. While your patient may actually be another ophthalmic assistant or even a physician, you should still explain what you are doing and what you want from the patient. Suppose you are taking a vertex distance. Tell the test patient the same thing you tell your patients in the office: "I need to measure the distance between your eye and the back of this lens. This is important so your glasses will be lined up correctly. See this little foot? It rests against your eyelid. So just close both eyes and keep them closed until I tell you. You'll feel this against your lid, but there won't be any pressure. Go ahead and close your eyes . . . I'm going to rest the instrument against your lid now . . . okay, all done!"

If you make a mistake or begin to have a hard time, just stop and take a deep breath or two. Above all else, keep your perspective. One time when I served as proctor, the candidate became frustrated and was verbally rude to the patient. That's inexcusable. If you're having problems, just tell the proctor that you want to begin that task again. (You see again why I advised you to perform the quicker, easier tasks first!)

When you write your answers on the answer sheet, be sure to double-check yourself. Make sure you are giving the information asked for. Make sure you are writing the answer in the proper space. And make sure of the numbers you write down. It would be a shame to fail a task because you transferred the wrong number from the instrument to the sheet.

Even though you're probably a little nervous, be sure to remember your manners. The proctors and test patients gave up their day off to help you. Be sure to thank them before leaving the room.

Bibliography

Adams AJ, Verdon WA, Spivey BE. Color vision. In: Tasman W, Jaeger EA, eds. *Duane's Ophthalmology* on CD-ROM. Philadelphia, Pa: Lippincott-Raven Publishers; 1996.

Appleton B. *Clinical Optics*. Thorofare, NJ: SLACK Incorporated; 1990.

Becker RA. Hypertension and arteriolsclerosis. In: Tasman W, Jaeger EA, eds. *Duane's Ophthalmology* on CD-ROM. Philadelphia, Pa: Lippincott-Raven Publishers; 1996.

Benes SC, McKinney K, Sanders LC, Miller M, Moberg M. *Advanced Ophthalmic Diagnostics and Therapeutics*. Thorofare, NJ: SLACK Incorporated; 1992.

Benson WE. An introduction to color vision. In: Tasman W, Jaeger EA, eds. *Duane's Ophthalmology* on CD-ROM. Philadelphia, Pa: Lippincott-Raven Publishers; 1996.

Bittinger M. *General Medical Knowledge for Eyecare Paraprofessionals*. Thorofare, NJ: SLACK Incorporated; 1999.

Blair B, Appleton B, Garber G, Crowe M, Alven M. *Opticianry, Ocularistry and Ophthalmic Technology*. Thorofare, NJ: SLACK Incorporated; 1990.

Borover WA. *Opticiany: The Practice and the Art. Vol. II – The Science of Opticianry*. Chula Vista, Calif: Gracie Enterprises, Inc; 1989.

Brown B. *The Low Vision Handbook*. Thorofare, NJ: SLACK Incorporated; 1997.

Brubaker RF. Tonometry. In: Tasman W, Jaeger EA, eds. *Duane's Ophthalmology* on CD-ROM. Philadelphia, Pa: Lippincott-Raven Publishers; 1996.

Burian HM, von Noorden GK. *Binocular Vision and Ocular Motility: Theory and Management of Strabismus*. St. Louis, Mo: CV Mosby Co; 1974.

Carlton J. *Frames and Lenses*. Thorofare, NJ: SLACK Incorporated. In press.

Cassin B. Classification and characteristics of eso deviations. In: Scott WE, D'Agostino DD, Lennarson LW. *Orthoptics and Ocular Examination Techniques*. Baltimore, Md: Williams & Wilkins; 1983.

Cassin B, ed. *Fundamentals for Ophthalmic Technical Personnel*. Philadelphia, Pa: WB Saunders; 1995.

Cassin B, McDavid D, Shamis D. Eye disorders. In: Cassin B, ed. *Fundamentals for Ophthalmic Technical Personnel*. Philadelphia, Pa: WB Saunders; 1995.

Choplin N, Edwards R. *Visual Fields*. Thorofare, NJ: SLACK Incorporated; 1998.

Choplin NT, Edwards RP. *Visual Field Testing With the Humphrey Field Analyzer*. Thorofare, NJ: SLACK Incorporated; 1995.

Cinotti AA, Kolker RH. *Ophthalmic Pharmacology. Home Study Course—Advanced Series*. Washington, DC: The American Association of Ophthalmology; 1968.

Coppinger JM, Maio M, Miller K. *Ophthalmic Photography*. Thorofare, NJ: SLACK Incorporated; 1988.

Creager JG, Black JG, Davison VE. *Microbiology: Principles & Applications*. Englewood Cliffs, NJ: Prentice Hall; 1990.

Cunningham D. *Clinical Ocular Photography*. Thorofare, NJ: SLACK Incorporated; 1998.

D'Agostino DD. Physiology of eye movements. In: Scott WE, D'Agostino DD, Lennarson LW, eds. *Orthoptics and Ocular Examination Techniques*. Baltimore, Md: Williams & Wilkins; 1983.

DuBois L. *Basic Procedures*. Thorofare, NJ: SLACK Incorporated; 1998.

Duvall B, Kershner RM. *Ophthalmic Medications and Pharmacology*. Thorofare, NJ: SLACK Incorporated; 1998.

Duvall B, Werner E, Lens A. *Cataract and Glaucoma for Eyecare Paraprofessionals*. Thorofare, NJ: SLACK Incorporated; 1999.

Faye EE. Low vision. In: Tasman W, Jaeger EA, eds. *Duane's Ophthalmology* on CD-ROM. Philadelphia, Pa: Lippincott-Raven Publishers; 1996.

Fedukowicz HB, Stenson S. *External Infections of the Eye*. 3rd ed. East Norwalk, Conn: Appleton-Century-Crofts; 1985.

Flynn JT. Clinical evaluation of the patient with congenital nystagmus. In: Scott WE, D'Agostino DD, Lennarson LW. *Orthoptics and Ocular Examination Techniques*. Baltimore, Md: Williams & Wilkins; 1983.

Folberg R, Bernardino VB Jr. Pathologic correlates in ophthalmoscopy. In: Tasman W, Jaeger EA, eds. *Duane's Ophthalmology* on CD-ROM. Philadelphia, Pa: Lippincott-Raven Publishers; 1996.

Foster A. Patterns of blindness. In: Tasman W, Jaeger EA, eds. *Duane's Ophthalmology* on CD-ROM. Philadelphia, Pa: Lippincott-Raven Publishers; 1996.

Garber N. Low vision. In: Scott WE, D'Agostino DD, Lennarson LW. *Orthoptics and Ocular Examination Techniques*. Baltimore, Md: Williams & Wilkins; 1983.

Garber N. *Visual Field Examination*. Thorofare, NJ: SLACK Incorporated; 1988.

Gayton JL, Ledford JR. *The Crystal Clear Guide to Sight for Life*. Lancaster, Pa: Starburst Publishers; 1996.

Ginsberg SP. Diseases and treatment of the vitreous and retina. In: Rhode SJ, Ginsberg SP, eds. *Ophthalmic Technology: A Guide for the Eye Care Assistant*. New York, NY: Raven Press; 1987.

Glaser JS. Topical diagnosis: prechiasmal visual pathways. In: Tasman W, Jaeger EA, eds. *Duane's Ophthalmology* on CD-ROM. Philadelphia, Pa: Lippincott-Raven Publishers; 1996.

Greenwald MJ, Parks MM. Amblyopia. In: Tasman W, Jaeger EA, eds. *Duane's Ophthalmology* on CD-ROM. Philadelphia, Pa: Lippincott-Raven Publishers; 1996.

Greenwald MJ, Parks MM. Treatment of amblyopia. In: Tasman W, Jaeger EA, eds. *Duane's Ophthalmology* on CD-ROM. Philadelphia, Pa: Lippincott-Raven Publishers; 1996.

Guyton DL. Automated clinical refraction. In: Tasman W, Jaeger EA, eds. *Duane's Ophthalmology* on CD-ROM. Philadelphia, Pa: Lippincott-Raven Publishers; 1996.

Gwin N. *Overview of Ocular Disorders*. Thorofare, NJ: SLACK Incorporated; 1999.

Hansen VC. *A Systematic Approach to Strabismus*. Thorofare, NJ: SLACK Incorporated; 1998.

Hargis-Greenshields L, Sims L. *Emergencies in Eyecare*. Thorofare, NJ: SLACK Incorporated; 1999.

Hoffman J. *Quick Reference Glossary of Eyecare Terminology*. 2nd ed. Thorofare, NJ: SLACK Incorporated; 1998.

Hunter DG, West CE. *Last Minute Optics*. Thorofare, NJ: SLACK Incorporated; 1996.

Johnson CA. Evaluation of visual function. In: Tasman W, Jaeger EA, eds. *Duane's Ophthalmology* on CD-ROM. Philadelphia, Pa: Lippincott-Raven Publishers; 1996.

Katz M. The human eye as an optical system. In: Tasman W, Jaeger EA, eds. *Duane's Ophthalmology* on CD-ROM. Philadelphia, Pa: Lippincott-Raven Publishers; 1996.

Kendall CJ. *Ophthalmic Echography*. Thorofare, NJ: SLACK Incorporated; 1990.

Kumar V, Cotran RS, Robbins SL. *Basic Pathology*. 5th ed. Philadelphia, Pa: WB Saunders; 1992.

Laney MD. Visual fields. In: Rhode SJ, Ginsberg SP, eds. *Ophthalmic Technology: A Guide for the Eye Care Assistant*. New York, NY: Raven Press; 1987.

Ledford JK. *Exercises in Refractometry*. Thorofare, NJ: SLACK Incorporated; 1990.

Ledford JK, Sanders VN. *The Slit Lamp Primer*. Thorofare, NJ: SLACK Incorporated; 1998.

Lennarson LW. Detection and measurement of strabismus. In: Scott WE, D'Agostino DD, Lennarson LW. *Orthoptics and Ocular Examination Techniques*. Baltimore, Md: Williams & Wilkins; 1983.

Lens A. *Optics, Retinoscopy, and Refractometry*. Thorofare, NJ: SLACK Incorporated; 1999.

Lens A, Langley T, Nemeth SC, Shea C. *Ocular Anatomy and Physiology*. Thorofare, NJ: SLACK Incorporated; 1999.

Lessell S, Lessell IM, Glaser JS. Topical diagnosis: retrochiasmal visual pathways and higher cortical function. In: Tasman W, Jaeger EA, eds. *Duane's Ophthalmology* on CD-ROM. Philadelphia, Pa: Lippincott-Raven Publishers; 1996.

McKenney SG. Binocular vision. In: Scott WE, D'Agostino DD, Lennarson LW, eds. *Orthoptics and Ocular Examination Techniques*. Baltimore, Md: Williams & Wilkins; 1983.

Migdal C. Primary open-angle glaucoma. In: Tasman W, Jaeger EA, eds. *Duane's Ophthalmology* on CD-ROM. Philadelphia, Pa: Lippincott-Raven Publishers; 1996.

Nemeth SC, Shea CA. *Medical Sciences for the Ophthalmic Assistant*. Thorofare, NJ: SLACK Incorporated; 1988.

Parks MM. Binocular vision. In: Tasman W, Jaeger EA, eds. *Duane's Ophthalmology* on CD-ROM. Philadelphia, Pa: Lippincott-Raven Publishers; 1996.

Parks MM. Monofixation syndrome. In: Tasman W, Jaeger EA, eds. *Duane's Ophthalmology* on CD-ROM. Philadelphia, Pa: Lippincott-Raven Publishers; 1996.

Parks MM, Mitchell PR. Dissociated vertical deviations. In: Tasman W, Jaeger EA, eds. *Duane's Ophthalmology* on CD-ROM. Philadelphia, Pa: Lippincott-Raven Publishers; 1996.

Parrish RK. *An Introduction to Visual Optics*. Rochester, Minn: American Academy of Ophthalmology and Otolaryngology; 1972.

Pavan-Langston D, ed. *Manual of Ocular Diagnosis and Therapy*. 2nd ed. Boston, Mass: Little, Brown, and Co; 1985.

Pickett K. *Overview of Ocular Surgery and Surgical Counseling*. Thorofare, NJ: SLACK Incorporated; 1999.

Raab EL. Exodeviations. In: Scott WE, D'Agostino DD, Lennarson LW, eds. *Orthoptics and Ocular Examination Techniques*. Baltimore, Md: Williams & Wilkins; 1983.

Rhode S. Refractometry. In: Rhode SJ, Ginsberg SP, eds. *Ophthalmic Technology: A Guide for the Eye Care Assistant*. New York, NY: Raven Press; 1987.

Rhode S. The electroretinogram and electro-oculogram. In: Rhode SJ, Ginsberg SP, eds. *Ophthalmic Technology: A Guide for the Eye Care Assistant*. New York, NY: Raven Press; 1987.

Rigillo CD, Maguire JI. Indocyanine green angiography. In: Tasman W, Jaeger EA, eds. *Duane's Ophthalmology* on CD-ROM. Philadelphia, Pa: Lippincott-Raven Publishers; 1996.

Ross FC. *Introductory Microbiology*. Columbus, Ohio: Charles E. Merrill Publishing Co; 1983.

Sabates FN. Applied laser optics: techniques for retinal laser surgery. In: Tasman W, Jaeger EA, eds. *Duane's Ophthalmology* on CD-ROM. Philadelphia, Pa: Lippincott-Raven Publishers; 1996.

Sassani JW. Glaucoma. In: Tasman W, Jaeger EA, eds. *Duane's Ophthalmology* on CD-ROM. Philadelphia, Pa: Lippincott-Raven Publishers; 1996.

Schechter RJ. Optics of intraocular lenses. In: Tasman W, Jaeger EA, eds. *Duane's Ophthalmology* on CD-ROM. Philadelphia, Pa: Lippincott-Raven Publishers; 1996.

Scott WE, D'Agostino DD, Lennarson LW. *Orthoptics and Ocular Examination Techniques*. Baltimore, Md: Williams & Wilkins; 1983.

Stamper RL, Sanghvi SS. Intraocular pressure: measurement, regulation, and flow relationships. In: Tasman W, Jaeger EA, eds. *Duane's Ophthalmology* on CD-ROM. Philadelphia, Pa: Lippincott-Raven Publishers; 1996.

Stein HA, Slatt BJ, Stein RM. *The Ophthalmic Assistant*. 6th ed. St. Louis, Mo: Mosby; 1994.

Stevens G Jr. Anatomy and physiology of the extraocular muscles. In: Rhode SJ, Ginsberg SP, eds. *Ophthalmic Technology: A Guide for the Eye Care Assistant*. New York, NY: Raven Press; 1987.

Van Boemel GB. *Special Skills and Techniques*. Thorofare, NJ: SLACK Incorporated; 1999.

Vaughan DG, Asbury T, Riordan-Eva P. *General Ophthalmology*. 13th ed. Norwalk, Conn: Appleton & Lange; 1992.

Waltersdorff RL. Microbiology: laboratory methods in diagnosing ocular infections. In: Rhode SJ, Ginsberg SP, eds. *Ophthalmic Technology: A Guide for the Eye Care Assistant*. New York, NY: Raven Press; 1987.

Wang FM. Perinatal ophthalmology. In: Tasman W, Jaeger EA, eds. *Duane's Ophthalmology* on CD-ROM. Philadelphia, Pa: Lippincott-Raven Publishers; 1996.

Wilson FM, Wilson FM II. Postoperative uveitis. In: Tasman W, Jaeger EA, eds. *Duane's Ophthalmology* on CD-ROM. Philadelphia, Pa: Lippincott-Raven Publishers; 1996.

Wong PC, Dickens CJ, Hoskins HD Jr. The developmental glaucomas. In: Tasman W, Jaeger EA, eds. *Duane's Ophthalmology* on CD-ROM. Philadelphia, Pa: Lippincott-Raven Publishers; 1996.

Printed in the United States
by Baker & Taylor Publisher Services